THE ROMANTIC STORY OF SCENT

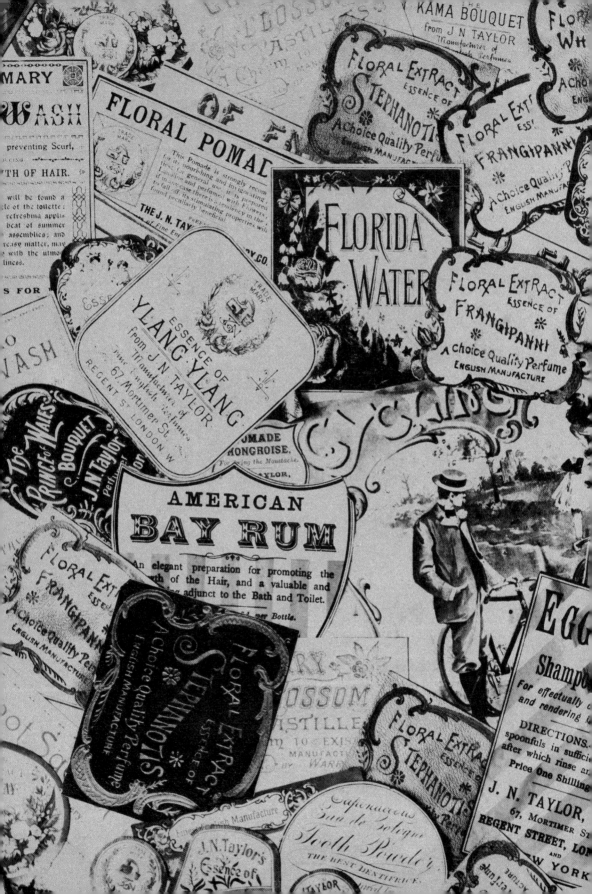

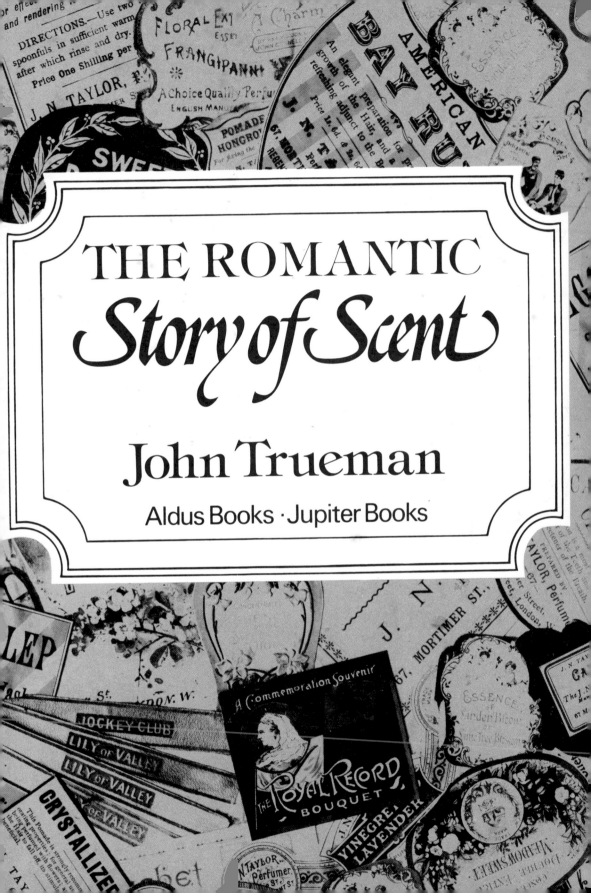

THE ROMANTIC
Story of Scent

John Trueman

Aldus Books · Jupiter Books

Conceived and designed by
Parkshot Paper Products

ISBN 0 904041 02 6

© 1975 Aldus Books Limited and Parkshot Paper Products Manufacturing Limited

First published in 1975 by Aldus Books Limited,
17 Conway Street, Fitzroy Square, London W1P 6BS.
Distributed by Jupiter Books,
167 Hermitage Road, Harringay, London N4 1LZ.

Printed and bound in the United Kingdom by
Tinling (1973) Ltd., Prescot, Merseyside.

CONTENTS

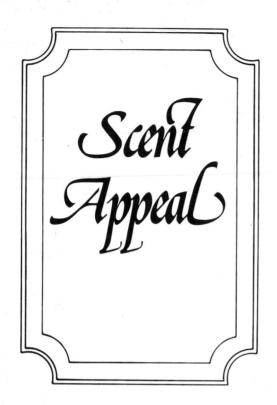

Scent Appeal

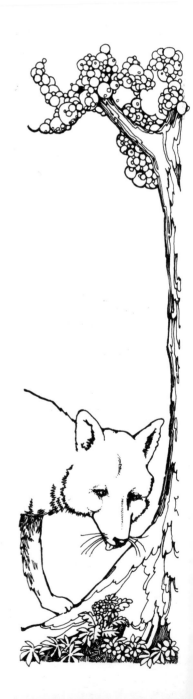

Man is the supreme example of the non-specialist animal. Physically, he does nothing exceptionally well. He is neither particularly fast nor particularly strong. And, by animal standards, none of his five senses is particularly acute. He gets his best marks for his eyesight. With his binocular vision and his upright stance, he is basically a 'seeing' animal. We even say 'I see' when we mean 'I understand'. Secondarily, he depends upon his hearing. He relies very little on his sense of smell – rather surprisingly, because smells are always with him. He cannot – because he has to breathe – close his nose to smells as he can his eyes and ears to sights and sounds. In company with monkeys, apes, and most birds he has a very poor sense of smell. Dogs, cats, and many other mammals use and depend upon their noses to a much greater extent. They are more sensitive to smell than man, and they extract much more information from the scent of their surroundings.

A bloodhound can detect the scent trace of a particular person in a room long after he or she has left it. A fox can sniff a tree and not only tell that another fox has been there, he can tell which fox and what it had for its last meal. A salmon can smell its way home over vast distances. It depends mainly on its sense of smell to enable it to navigate to its place of birth for spawning – it recognizes a specific combination of scents from its native river. A male butterfly can detect the scent of a female several miles away – even though she carries less than one ten-thousandth of a milligram of her special perfume and exudes only a minute proportion of it into the air at any moment. Beside such feats as these, man's capacity to smell is rudimentary.

Yet, we all have large, protruding noses. Why are they comparatively so inefficient? The answer is that the primary function of the human nose is to channel pre-heated, filtered air to the lungs. Smell is very much a secondary function. The olfactory cells – the scent detectors – occupy only a very limited area of the mucous membranes of the nose. There are some five million of these cells, situated right at the top of the nasal cavity. It sounds a lot, but, comparatively speaking, it is a very meagre ration. A dachshund has about 125 million olfactory cells and a German sheepdog has something like 220 million. But even this does not account completely for our relative insensitivity to scent. The sheepdog's sense of smell is not, as we should expect, 44 times as acute as man's. It is roughly a million times more acute. So not only do we have relatively few olfactory cells; those that we have are not as efficient as they might be. It seems that early man – because, by standing up on his hind legs, he had given himself the benefit of a wider field of vision – came to rely almost entirely on his eyesight. He relied on seeing his approaching predator or enemy, on navigating by visual landmarks, and on recognizing his mate by her looks. So his sense of smell atrophied.

As far as we know, man has never used his own scent, as many other territorial animals do, to mark out his territory. Antelope, for example, mark twigs with a strong-smelling substance secreted in glands on their faces. The roebuck has a similar gland on its forehead, which it rubs against branches to deposit its scent. Hamsters use their flank glands to put a fence of scent around their territories. Badgers use their anal glands. Voles squirt their glandular secretions on to the soles of their feet and trample their scent into the earth as they walk their boundaries.

This sort of behaviour seems never to have occurred in man. He has never made much use of his own body odours. This is partly because he appears to have lost his smell as well as his sense of smell. The anthropologist Dr Louis S. B. Leakey has suggested that early man owed his survival to his distinctive body odour, which was so rank that it turned the stomachs of predatory animals. Because of this they found him uneatable and left him alone until he had time to learn to protect himself by the use of weapons. Then his unpleasant body smell, having no practical use, began to disappear. This may, or may not, be what happened; it is certainly true that we have lost our original strong animal odour.

Nevertheless, we still smell – mainly through our sweat. If you walk barefoot, every footprint you leave is impregnated with about four-billionths of a gram of odorous sweat substance. It is a tiny amount, but a

Today, the world of scent is being rediscovered. The trail-blazers and pioneer explorers were the young. They were the first to realize that our sense of smell can be educated to be as receptive to pleasures and experiences as our other senses. They have learned to surround themselves with scent on a scale that the Western world has not known for hundreds, perhaps thousands, of years. They use scents with the same freedom as did the peoples of some ancient nations long before the birth of Christ. But they have an advantage over those earlier peoples. Living in the latter part of the 20th century, they are able to enjoy scented products in a variety never before known. Some of the scented pleasure toys now available to them are shown in THE SCENT SCENE *overleaf* and are listed in the key to the illustration on page 10.

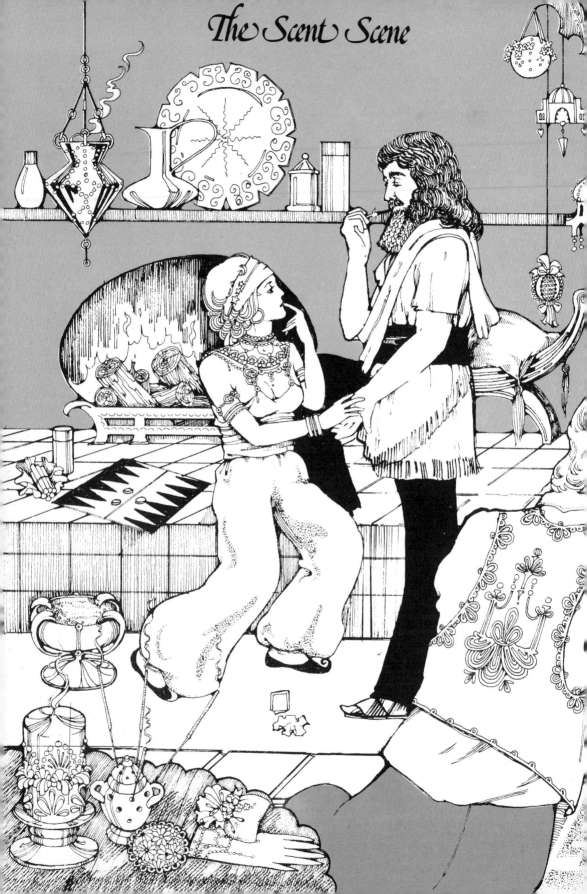

The Scent Scene

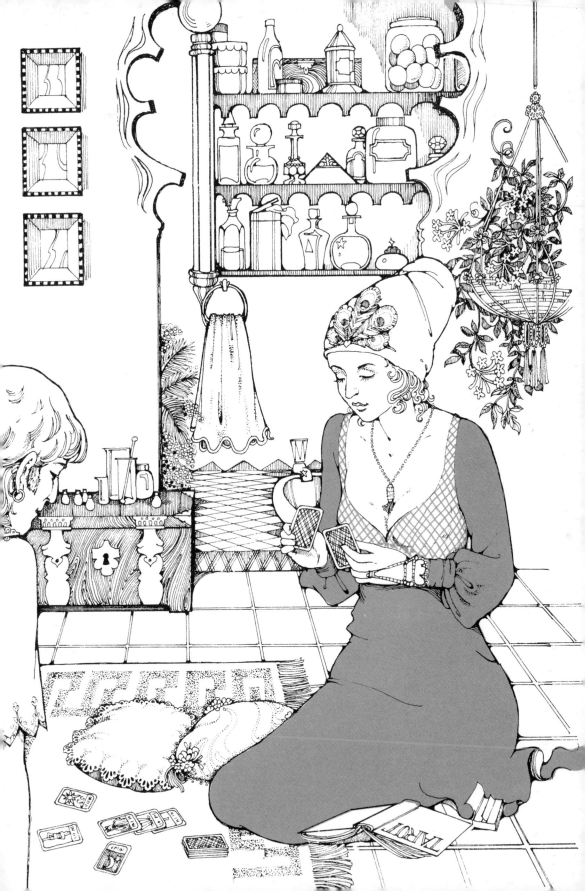

The back-to-scent experience is not just an inexplicable, easily dismissed fad. It is an end-result of many interwoven strands of deeply felt responses and reactions. One strand is the reaction against the destruction of our earth's resources, which has led to a rediscovered feeling for the value of natural things and, by extension, to a desire to enjoy simple, natural delights. Hence the recent popularity, in the world of scent, of natural flower fragrances. Another strand is a revulsion against the materialist propaganda machine and a feeling that it is better to surround oneself with sensuous pleasures that arouse the imagination than passively to be entertained by the media. Better to switch oneself on than to switch the television on. Hence the use of scent in a larger number of experimental ways. Yet another strand is the search for some kind of spiritual belief now that Western society has become de-Christianized. That search led to the East. The hippy trail to India in the 1960s pioneered it, and the return cargo of the hippy trail included the fashion, music, art — and scents — of the East. Eastern fragrances, such as patchouli, musk, and sandalwood, are — like backgammon and Tarot cards— thus the not-so-trivial by-products of a spiritual quest.

1 *Scent Scenes* — hollow picture frames, with vents at the back, serving as holders for sweet-scented pot-pourris
2 Censers for perfuming the house
3 Turkish copperware
4 Ready-to-use powder for making pot-pourris the easy way
5 Pottery and laminated-board pomanders filled with pot-pourri
6 Splash-on colognes
7 Eau de Cologne tissue canister
8 Scented soap
9 Log fire of scented pear and apple wood
10 Fashionably dressed man with 'spade' beard and clothing copied, in part, from styles worn in ancient Assyria
11 Do-it-yourself scent-making kit
12 Conical hat fashioned in the style worn by men in ancient Assyria
13 Indonesian clove and incense cigarettes
14 Backgammon
15 Dish containing pot-pourri
16 Pantaloons
17 *Scented Shoe Cosmetic* — self-shining wax-impregnated pads for cleaning and scenting leather shoes
18 Sandalwood box
19 Pot-pourri locket
20 Scented gloves and leather jerkin
21 Lavender- and herb-filled cushions
22 Malayan dress
23 Scented candles
24 Joss sticks
25 Sachets for scenting clothes
26 Pack of Tarot cards
27 Clove-scented cigarette papers

The Scent Scene

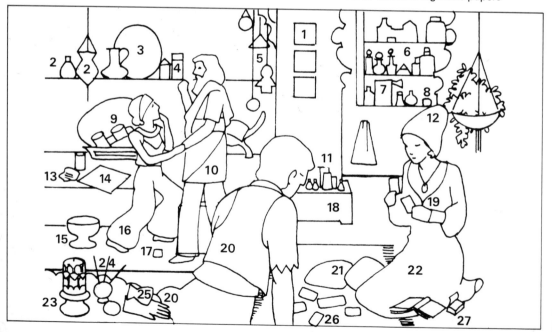

tracker dog will detect it with no difficulty at all. Indeed, a dog will be able to track you even if you wear Wellington boots; enough scent will penetrate the soles of the boot for the dog still to follow your trail. What is more, he will pick out your trail from other peoples'. We all smell differently. Even identical twins have different natural odours. This is because the scent we give off is not a single, pure one. It is the product of many different fatty acids and of the action of bacteria upon them. The possible permutations – in number, quantity, and inter-action – are so numerous that no two people have the same scent. Our odour is as individual to each of us as are our facial characteristics or our fingerprints.

Many attempts have been made to classify human smells. In his book *The Gilded Lily,* Terence McLaughlin notes that, according to a German student of the psychology of scent, 'very fair people, particularly the Scandinavian type of blond, have a skin odour similar to that of rancid butter mixed with decaying leather, redheads have a skin odour just like rancid butter mixed with catmint, while dark brunettes have a smell like decomposing goats'. A Frenchman, perhaps typically, was more gallant. According to Augustin Galopin, whose book *Le Parfum de la Femme* was published in Paris in 1866, redheads have the strongest smell of all women, brunettes are next, and blondes the most faintly scented. Redheads, and women with chestnut hair, smell of amber or of violets; brunettes have the scent of ebony; blondes have a more subtle odour of amber or of violets.

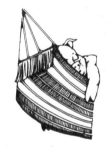

Galopin has brought us to the heart of the matter – which is, of course, the eroticism of scent. Throughout the animal kingdom scent plays an important part in courtship and in mating. Most of us have seen the effect that the scent of a bitch in season has on a dog. There is a reason for the dog's excitement. Many species of animals, especially those that have periods of heat, are known to possess substances, called pheromones, whose scent infallibly triggers the lust of the opposite sex. In pigs the pheromone is a hormone that the scientists have named androstenone. It is now available in aerosol form and is used by breeders to make the sow instantly ready for the boar. The pheromone has been isolated also from female monkeys, although its chemical make-up has not yet been unravelled. Whatever it is, it is irresistible to the male monkey.

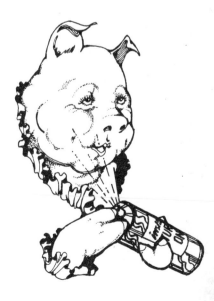

Do human males and females carry pheromones? Did they ever? The questions cannot yet be answered. But certainly scent plays a part in human love, even if usually on a more or less unconscious level. When we kiss we are performing an attenuated ceremony of greeting by smelling; in many primitive languages the word for 'kiss' or 'greet' is the same as that for 'smell'. Nonetheless, we would probably quickly be turned off if our loved one whispered 'I want to be smelled' rather than 'I want to be kissed'.

This is because we have pushed scent out of reality and into romance. Unlike other animals, man has the power of creative imagination and of introspection, and is able to savour his own emotional responses. So while scent became in practical terms less important to him, it became more important as a source of sensuous pleasure. When he no longer used his nose to smell out danger, he began relaxedly to enjoy the smell of flowers and the aroma of roasting meat. In this sensuous response to scent he is probably alone among the animals. In the words of one of the earliest English herbals, William Bullein's 16th-century *Bulwarke against Sickness:* 'Man only doth smell and take delight in the odours of flowers and sweet things'.

This romanticization has led to some curious paradoxes. One is that, although our sense of smell is, as we have seen, comparatively rudimentary, our emotional response to scent is acutely sensitive. 'Sweet scents,' wrote the poet Walter Savage Landor, 'are the sweet vehicles of still sweeter thoughts'. Almost every one of us can name a scent that for us recaptures a moment, an event, an experience. As Rudyard Kipling put it, 'Scents are surer than sights and sounds to make your heart-strings crack'. In a television programme broadcast in 1970, a group of railwaymen described their memories of the days of steam. Almost all of them remembered best a particular smell. One recalled the smell of the engine shed on a winter's morning, with the fires burning in the fire-boxes. But most of them agreed that their most vivid recollection was of the scent of apple blossom as they took their trains out of the industrial smog of the Midlands and came down into the fields and orchards of Worcestershire. Rupert Brooke, the poet of the First World War, remembered the scented flowers of a vicarage garden:

> *And in my flower beds, I think,*
> *Smile the carnation and the pink.*

Another English poet, Lord Tennyson, found in the scent of flowers a nostalgia for a lost age of innocence:

> *The smell of violets hidden in the green*
> *Pour'd back into my empty soul and frame*
> *The times when I remember to have been*
> *Joyful and free from blame.*

This makes it, again, odd that we are singularly short of words with which we can describe scents meaningfully to one another. We can describe colours easily enough. There are a variety of words to portray sounds, and we can at least describe tastes as either bitter or sweet. But odours we can describe only by analogy, hoping that our hearer's subjective impressions correspond with our own. We may say that something smells like violets, or that it has the perfume of strawberries or peaches. We can wax metaphorical, saying that something has a 'fresh' or a 'clean' smell. But how can a smell be 'clean'? It may seem even stranger to characterize a smell as 'big and round' or 'small and square'. But it may be

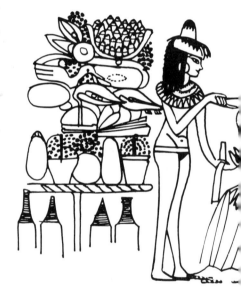

literally correct. No one knows how the olfactory cells in our noses work, but recently three American scientists put forward the theory that the cells operate not chemically but by recognizing the size and shape of the molecules of the substances presented to them. In the receptor cell there are sub-microscopically small apertures of various shapes and sizes, into which slot the equivalently shaped molecules. It is rather like the toddler's game of posting plastic shapes into a toy letter box. Spherical molecules register as the smell of camphor, discs as musk, 'tailed' discs as undifferentiated flowers, wedges as peppermint, and rods as ether. All smells are made up from these basic ingredients, rather as all colours can be made from the primary colours.

But the biggest paradox of all is the way in which we use scents today. We are all – men and women alike – artificially scented. Even those men who still do not use an after-shave lotion or a body-splash cologne must use a scented soap and probably a scented shaving cream – they are almost impossible to avoid. Women,

We have to go back to ancient Egypt to find scent used on the scale that it is beginning to reach again today. In this copy of a wall painting, of the 15th century B.C., from a tomb in Thebes, Egyptian women wear cooling cones of perfumed wax on their heads.

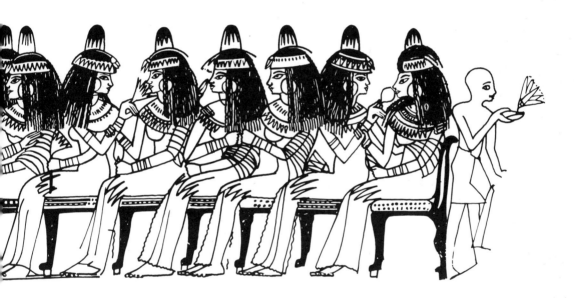

perhaps more deliberately than men, use artificial scents for a variety of reasons. Perfumes are, and have been for thousands of years, a necessary component of a woman's make-up kit.

A woman uses scent as she uses any other cosmetic, partly for social reasons – to announce her role in the community and to proclaim her conformity to the standards of her group. But she also uses it for sexual purposes, to attract the male. And this is certainly odd. Because she will have carefully washed away all her natural sexual odour. She will have inhibited its reappearance by applying antiperspirants and deodorants. Living in the 1970s, she may even use a vaginal deodorant. Then, having eliminated the residual feminine odours that evolution has permitted her to retain, she takes all the products of the perfumer's skill in order to replace her natural aromas with those that she thinks will make her more attractive to the male.

Her thinking is sound. Modern man has put his animal ancestors firmly behind him. He reacts to scents sophisticatedly and imaginatively. He prefers perfumes that trigger not his instincts but his emotions – partly, no doubt, because he is a social animal and, as a social animal, he has had to erect elaborate culture patterns around his courtship and mating. Animal odours are too direct for social man to cope with; the complex chemicals of a modern manufactured perfume are more effective and more to his taste.

The firm of Picot marketed a perfume called *Pagan*. Their advertisements said: '*Pagan* is for lovers. Don't wear it if you're only bluffing'. Allowing for the copy-writer's exaggeration, it was good advice. It is a fact of human cultural evolution that as an erotic 'releaser' a perfume like *Pagan* is more effective than the scent that nature gives to a woman's body.

What are these perfumes that please modern man's less refined nose and more fastidious mind? What ingredients go into them? Mostly, they are substances that have been known and used in perfumery for hundreds if not thousands of years. Many are obtained from plants. The scent that comes from a flower or herb is due to an essential oil carried in some part of the plant that gives it its particular aroma. The perfumer robs the plant of these oils – taking them from the petals of the rose, the jasmine, the violet, and the orange; from the leaves of a rock rose and a mint; from the fruits of the orange, the lemon, and the bergamot; from the wood itself of sandalwood and cedarwood. Other perfume-giving substances – such as ambergris, musk, castoreum, and civet – he takes from animals. Today he can also use synthetic materials – in the main the by-products of coal tar and petroleum. Some of these are man-made imitations of natural scents, others are the new inventions of the laboratory.

There are many thousands of these products available to the perfumer. A manufactured perfume may consist of a hundred or more different substances. Each has its separate identity, but each loses its identity as it is blended with its fellows to produce a composition as exciting to the nose as is a painting to the eyes or a piece of music to the ears.

It is these substances that we are now going to see – and smell.

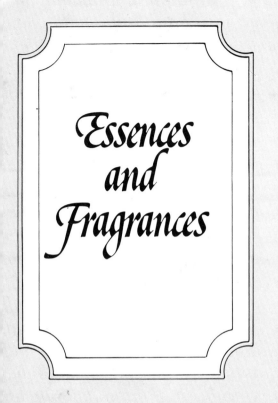

Essences
and
Fragrances

Any glamorously packed and romantically named perfume that you may buy in a shop is simply a mixture of a number of fragrant substances — sometimes natural, sometimes artificial — dissolved in an alcohol base. In this chapter we describe some of the most important of these substances, which are the raw materials of the perfumer.

But it is almost impossible to describe a fragrance in words. We can describe a smell only by comparing it with another smell. Often, this turns out to be a fairly meaningless operation. If we say that bergamot smells like rosemary, it is of no help to you if you have never smelled rosemary. Even if you have, to your nose the two substances may smell quite differently. Similarly, you may read that patchouli has an unpleasant, musty smell. Smell it for yourself and you may disagree. Patchouli may be the one scent that really turns you on. Scent impressions are subjective and only your nose can tell you what you like. In the event, the proof of the fragrance is in the smelling.

In this chapter, therefore, we have given you the smells. We have captured the scents of the substances we describe and printed them on paper.

On the jacket flaps of this book you will find 18 labels that correspond in shape, colour, and wording to the headings throughout this chapter. Each label may easily be peeled from the flap and placed in position covering the printed heading on the appropriate page of the book. Each is coated with adhesive and will stick permanently in its new position. Don't wet it, simply press it firmly down.

These labels are coated with an invisible film that consists of many millions of microscopically tiny capsules, each of which contains fragrance. It is as though we had filled billions of ping-pong balls with scent, scattered them thickly over many square miles of paper, and then magically shrunk the whole thing down to the size of a cigarette paper. In the coating on our labels, the ping-pong balls are microscopic capsules of gelatin; there are about 200 of them to an area the size of a pin head.

To release the fragrance, you simply scratch a tiny area of the label with your fingernail, thus breaking open some of the capsules.

Elsewhere in this book many more than 18 fragrances are, of course, mentioned. Here, we have had to be selective. Some fragrances we simply could not bring you. Saffron and frangipani, for example, both of which are of some historical interest, are no longer commercially available. Spikenard is almost impossible to obtain and, as its scent closely resembles that of lemon grass, we settled for lemon grass only. Myrrh was another candidate for inclusion, but its history so closely parallels that of frankincense that we decided to admit frankincense only. On the other hand, we have included an odd man out. We have re-created the ancient perfume of kyphi.

When we began the research and experiment that resulted in the micro-encapsulation of these scents, we used only genuine perfume essences derived from nature. But in the end we were forced to use some synthetics. Natural sandalwood and natural ambergris both refused to submit to encapsulation. We tried another formulation, using a mixture of natural and synthetic materials for both scents. Both failed. At the third attempt, with different proportions of the natural and synthetic materials, we succeeded in capturing the elusive sandalwood and ambergris scents. In much the same way, we found that natural lavender, vetivert, castoreum, and lemon grass all smelled rather jaded after encapsulation. We have had to fortify all these with synthetics. For the rose label we first used genuine Bulgarian attar of roses, but the soaring, sky-high price of this essence forced us to replace it by a synthetic. In our musk formulation there is no natural musk at all. Our synthetic imitation is, however, almost indistinguishable from the real thing. Natural cyprinum is no longer available; again, we had to match it by using synthetics. The clove, patchouli, and vetivert labels, however, all encapsulate only genuine, natural, unadulterated essences.

15

Jasmine

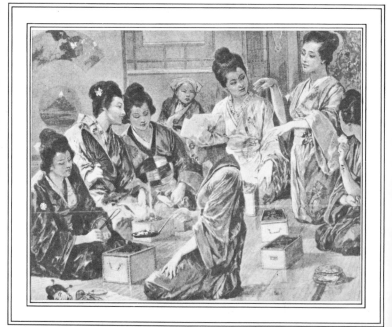

To the perfumer, the petals of the jasmine are as precious as those of the rose. Jasmine is an ingredient of almost every fine perfume.

The jasmine used in perfumery is obtained from the white jasmine, *Jasminum officinale,* a native of Persia and Kashmir. White jasmine is today grown commercially in Egypt, Italy, Corsica, Algeria, and Morocco, but the blossoms most valued by the perfumer are those cultivated around the town of Grasse in France.

Grasse is the centre of the French perfume industry. In nearby fields grow thousands of jasmine bushes, whose blossoms are gathered in July and August and again in October. It is this second flowering that produces jasmine of the highest fragrance. The flowers are at their most highly scented at dawn, and so it is at dawn that women and children gather the blossoms, transferring them into wicker baskets in which they are rushed to the factories.

Essence of jasmine for the perfumer's use is made from the blossoms by the process known as 'enfleurage', an old and costly method of extraction in which the scent of the petals is absorbed by cold purified fat (usually lard or suet), washed from the fat by alcohol, and finally separated from the alcohol by distillation.

Right: Kama, the Hindu god of love, aims an arrow at a young girl. In Hindu mythology, Kama was said to have had five arrows, each of which was tipped with the blossom of a fragrant flower and each of which pierced the heart of its victim through one of the five senses. The jasmine – known in India as 'Moonlight of the Grove' – was one of the five flowers of Kama. Jasmine has been held in reverence by other religions also; it appears often in paintings as a symbol of hope, happiness, and love.

Right: the game of Guess the Perfume. Incense parties were a popular amusement for well-to-do Japanese women in the early years of this century. Each player was provided with a miniature furnace – a small wooden box of sand on which burned a charcoal fire. The object of the game was to identify the perfumes in the incense each player was burning. Jasmine would certainly have been one of the mystery scents; it was a favourite perfume of the Japanese – and of the Chinese, who were fond of jasmine-scented tea.

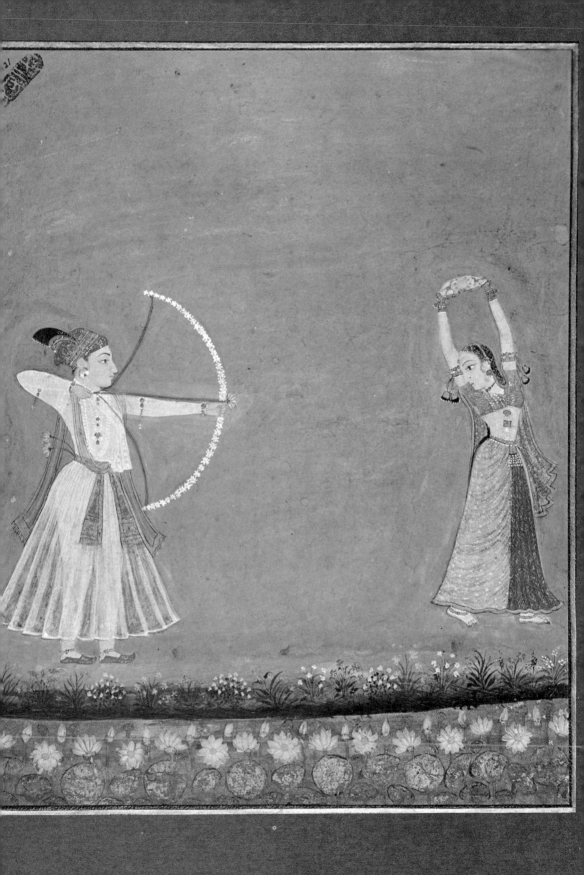

Kyphi

Kyphi is an invention of the ancient Egyptians, who made it to burn as incense, believing that it would waft their prayers more swiftly and more fragrantly to the gods. It was a mixture, according to the Greek biographer Plutarch, of sixteen scented herbs and resins – including myrrh, henna, cinnamon, juniper, honey, and raisins – all of which were steeped in wine. From another Greek writer, Democritus, who added two more ingredients, spikenard and saffron, we learn that the whole concoction was beaten up into a paste and then allowed to solidify.

Kyphi was a sacred perfume. Its preparation was a religious ritual, and it was burned at evening in the temples of Egypt as a fragrant offering to the setting sun. But its pleasures were not only for the gods. Kyphi was used in Egyptian homes, where also it was customarily burned at night. Plutarch says of it that it would induce sleep and brighten dreams, because it was made of 'those things that delight most in the night'.

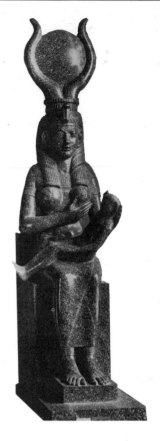

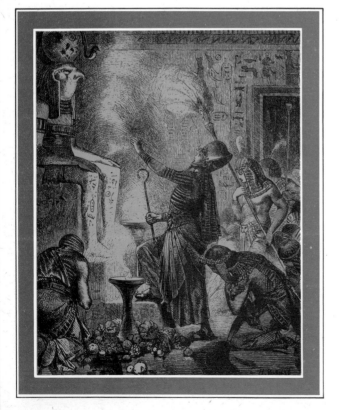

Above: the Egyptian goddess Isis, who reassembled the body of her husband Osiris after it had been torn into fourteen parts and scattered throughout Egypt. She gave Osiris immortality by anointing his body with precious oils and thus was the originator of the Egyptian rites of embalmment in which kyphi played so important a part.

Left: the pharaoh Akhenaton in the temple. The air is heavy with ascending incense as the sacred perfume burns at the feet of the god.

Right: feeding the sacred ibis in the great temple of Karnak. The ibis represented Thoth, the Egyptian god of wisdom and of the moon, and it is to him, rather than the birds, that the offering both of food and of perfume is being made.

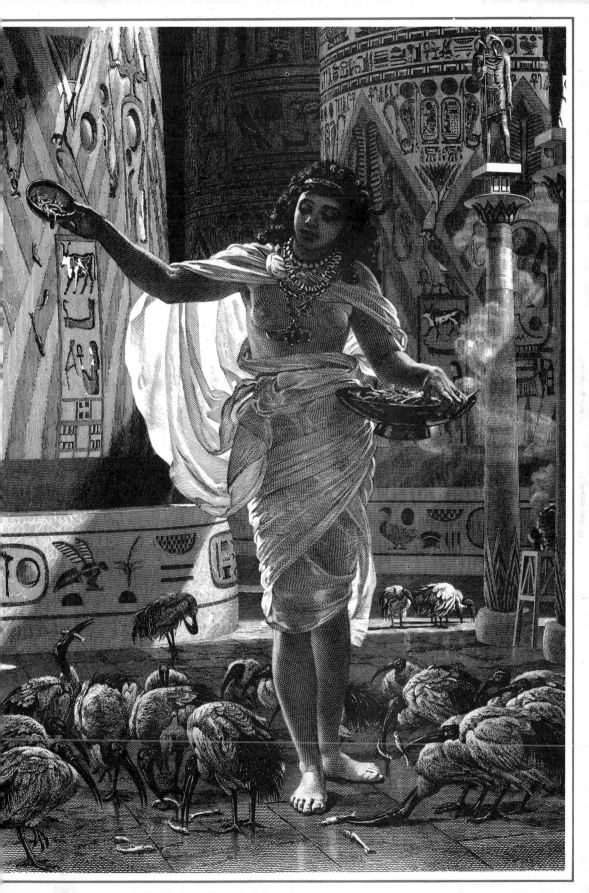

Sandalwood

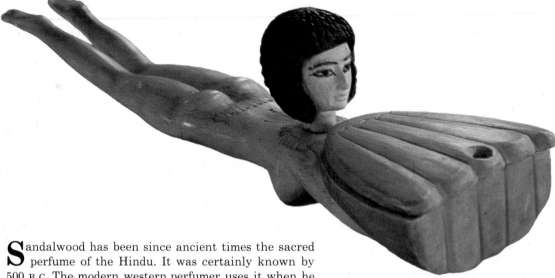

Below: an ancient Egyptian cosmetic box carved from sandalwood.

Sandalwood has been since ancient times the sacred perfume of the Hindu. It was certainly known by 500 B.C. The modern western perfumer uses it when he wishes to give an exotic, eastern flavour to a perfume and also values it as a 'fixative'. A fixative is what makes a perfume long-lasting; it is an ingredient that has the power of equalizing the rate of evaporation of all the other ingredients, so that the perfume's fragrance remains unaltered right up to the end of its life.

Sandalwood is obtained from the white wood of *Santalum album*, a parasitic tree that attaches itself to the roots of other trees and draws nourishment from them so successfully that it can grow to a height of over forty feet. The tree once grew in vast numbers in the dense forests of northern India, Burma, and China. But, because it is one of the few woods immune to attack by the all-devouring white ants that infested these areas, it was cut down in such numbers for use in building that it became scarce in its homelands and sandalwood had to be imported from Indonesia and the islands of the Timor Sea. Today the best quality wood for the perfumer comes from Mysore in India and from Australia.

It takes about a hundredweight of sandalwood chippings to yield thirty ounces of attar of sandalwood. The attar is often used in combination with attar of roses. It is a custom in Burma for women, on the last day of the year, to sprinkle passers-by with a mixture of rose water and essence of sandalwood to wash away the sins of the year.

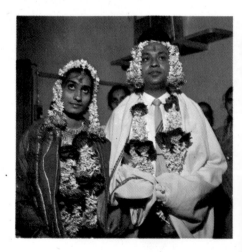

Above: a Hindu marriage ceremony. Sandalwood still plays an important part in Hindu marriages. It is burned on the sacred fire within the marriage tent so that its fumes surround the bridal couple.

20

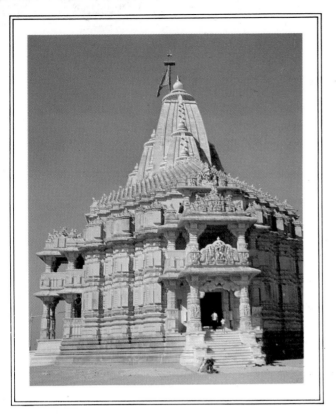

Left: the temple at Somnath, India, whose gates – like those of many other Hindu temples – were made of precious sandalwood. To Hindus sandalwood is the most important incense. During religious festivals for the god Vishnu alms are collected in exchange for sticks of scented sandalwood.

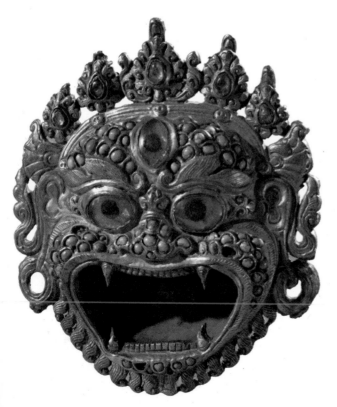

Left: a portable incense burner, about 4 ins. high, from Tibet, made of gilded copper inlaid with precious stones. Incense is used in all Tibetan religious ceremonies and this portable incense burner would be used daily to keep away evil spirits. A priest would also place it at the feet of the dead so that the soul might be wafted upwards to heaven in the perfume of the incense.

Cyprinum

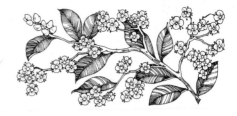

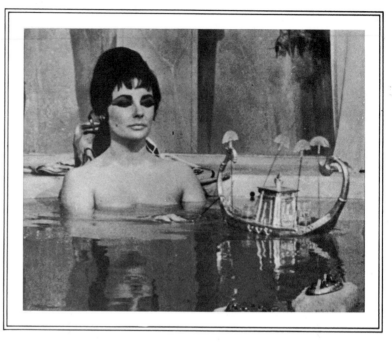

Elizabeth Taylor in the name part of one Hollywood version of the story of Cleopatra. The real Cleopatra was no great beauty, although she seems to have had no lack of sex appeal. Her seduction of Antony was helped by a lavish use of perfume, with which she was notoriously extravagant in an age when the rich at least used perfumes with careless abandon. It is recorded that on one occasion she used unguents to the enormous value of 400 denarii simply to soften and perfume her hands.

Every part of the henna plant, *Lawsonia inermis*, is perfumed. Under its other name of camphire the plant was one of the 'odorous bushy shrubs' placed by Milton in the Garden of Eden. It is thought to have been used as a hedge plant in the Hanging Gardens of Babylon. It can still be seen forming windbreaks around the vineyards of the Middle East, a function that it has been performing since ancient times. 'My beloved', proclaimed the writer of the Song of Solomon, 'is unto me as a cluster of camphire in the vineyards of En-gedi'.

The flower of the henna plant gives us a heady, long-lasting perfume called cyprinum. Cyprinum is a green-coloured, heavy scent, although the flower it comes from is white and delicate. Mahomed held the henna's scented flowers in high esteem; he called them 'the chief of the sweet-scented flowers of this world and the next.'

Mahomed also used henna to dye his beard. Mahomedan women used it to tint both their hair and their bodies. In this they followed the example of the women of ancient Egypt, who rubbed henna leaves on their cheeks and hands to give them a rouged look and who used a paste made from dried and powdered henna leaves to darken their hair.

Right: traditional henna body decoration. The henna plant is dried, pounded, and strained then mixed with water to produce a green, elastic substance. This is painted on to the skin with a pointed wooden stick. As the henna dries a mixture of lemon juice, sugar, pepper, and garlic is continually applied to prevent the henna flaking off. The depth and permanence of the resulting stain depends on the length of time the henna is left in place.

Overleaf: Cleopatra prepared to receive Antony aboard her barge. Its sails, dyed with the symbolic purple of royalty, would have been drenched with cyprinum and its hangings washed with scented waters. The canopy beneath which she sat was garlanded with roses, and slaves puffed towards her incense from bronze censers. Shakespeare has described the scene with matchless mastery:

Purple the sails, and so perfumed, that
The winds were love-sick with them . . . .

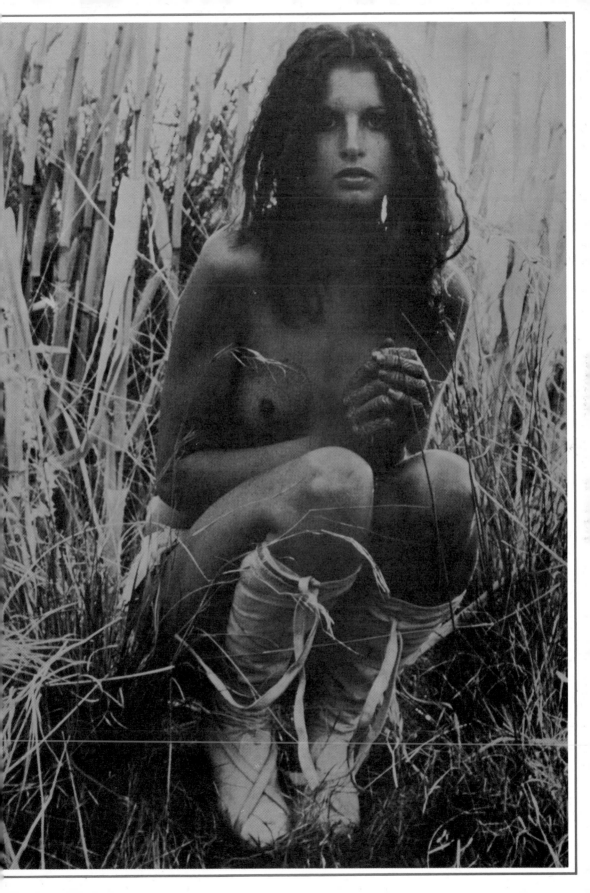

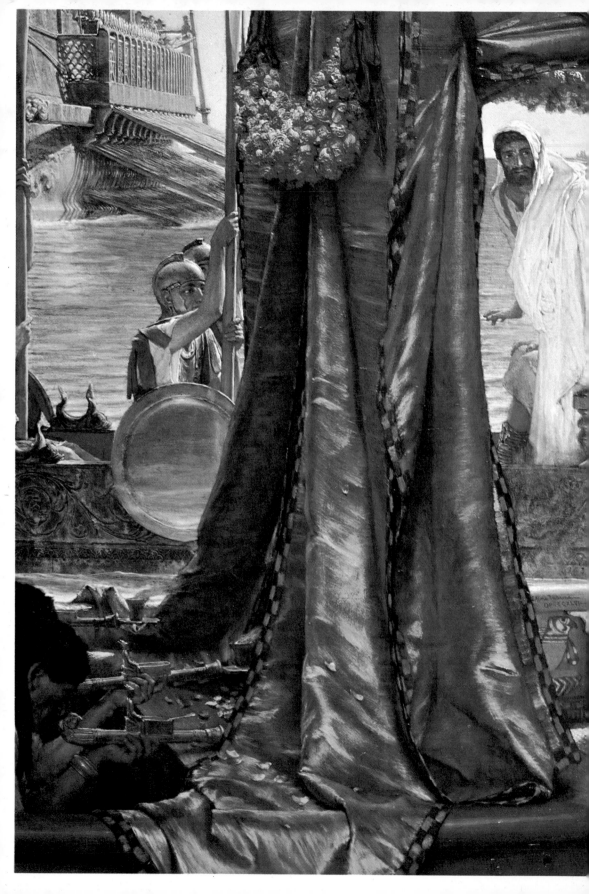

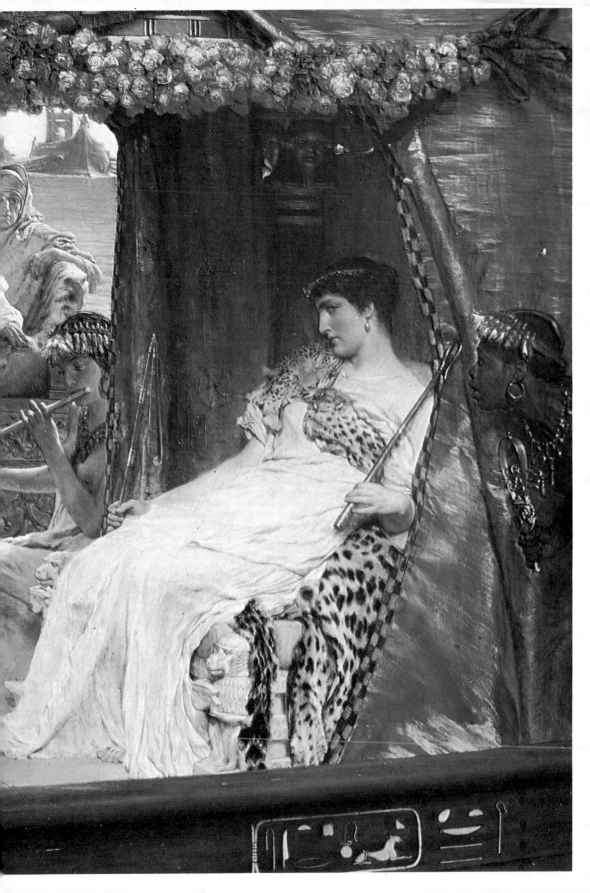

Musk

Musk is the most potent of all perfumes. Its sweet, penetrating scent is absorbed and retained by anything in its vicinity – even, it has been reported, polished steel. For this reason, the British East India Company, in the 19th century, refused to accept musk as a cargo on any ship that was also carrying tea. Musk is also the preferred aphrodisiac of the perfume world; it is thought to give any perfume an erotic 'lift' and to stimulate desire in those who wear it and those who inhale it.

Musk is an animal perfume. It is a glandular secretion of the musk deer, which lives in the dense forests just below the snow line in the Himalayas. Musk is obtained only from the male deer. It forms in a gland, or pod, about the size of a large walnut that grows between the flesh and the skin of the deer's abdomen. The pod can be reached through a hole in the animal's skin that is just big enough to take a man's little finger, and can be removed without harming the deer. The musk seems to be simply an accumulation of waste products in the animal's body. Indeed, the dung of the male deer – and only of the male – smells strongly of musk at most times of the year. But the musk is most abundant when the animal is in rut, which suggests that it plays some part in courtship and mating.

The pod is present at the deer's birth, but for the first two years or so of the animal's life the musk it contains is merely a milky liquid with an unpleasant stench. As the deer grows older, the musk increases in quantity and solidifies into grains.

How and when musk was discovered and how and when it was first used in perfumery we do not know. We find no record of it until about the turn of the sixth and seventh centuries A.D. By this time musk was among the precious spices and perfumes that Arab merchant ships – equipped with the new, efficient triangular sails and so able to voyage as far as India and China – were bringing back to the Mediterranean.

Musk became particularly popular in the Mahomedan world. In the Garden of Paradise, according to the Koran, the believer will be welcomed by beautiful houris created entirely of musk. But musk has always been popular, everywhere. In 1971 a craze for single-note perfumes that swept across the United States and spread to Britain centred upon musk. By 1974 that musk craze was over. But musk will certainly maintain its position as the preferred scent for lovers.

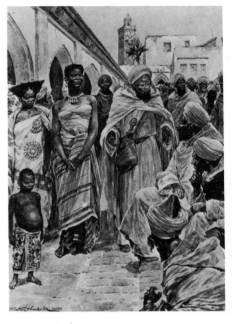

Above: the slave market in Marrakesh, Morocco, in 1905. Arab merchants had been trading in slaves for hundreds of years. They had long exported slaves and other merchandise to India and China in exchange for musk and other products of the East.

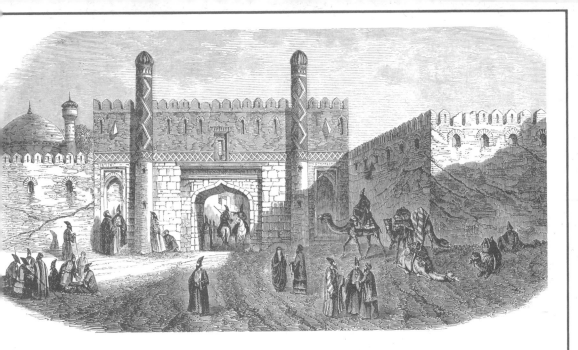

Above: the gate of the town of Tabriz in Iran. In the left background can be seen the minaret and dome of the Mosque of Zobiade. The followers of Mahomed valued musk above all other scents and they took advantage of its long-lasting properties by incorporating it in some of their buildings. Many of their mosques — including that at Tabriz — were built with mortar that had been mixed with musk. The mosques so built retained their pervasive aroma of musk for very long periods. It is even said with some exaggeration caused by wishful thinking, that the Mosque of Zobiade still smells of musk today.

Right: a pair of musk deer. The deer is about the size of a greyhound, measuring about two feet high at the shoulder. It is a nocturnal animal, its grey fur providing good night-time camouflage. Its protruding vampirish teeth are used to dig up the roots on which it lives. It may be this diet that produces the deer's unique scent.

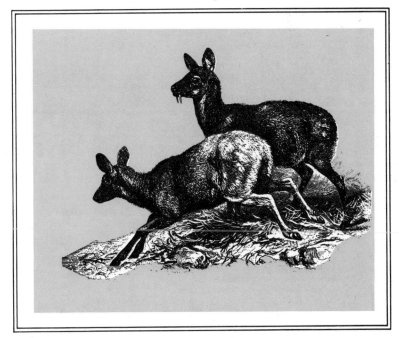

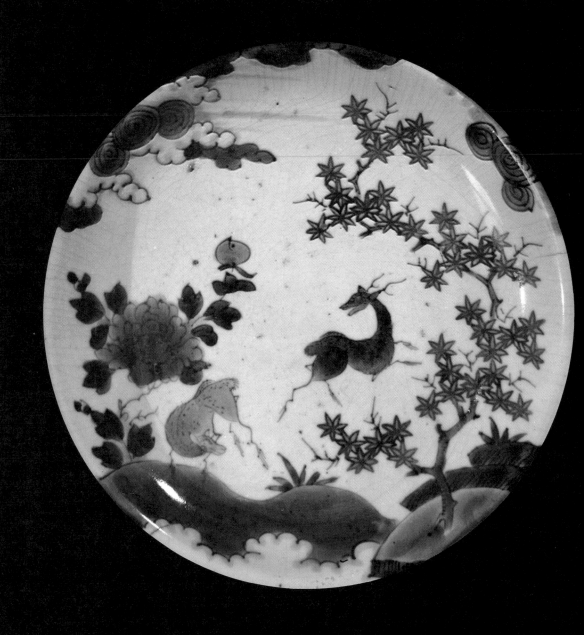

A Chinese plate depicting a graceful-looking musk deer. Musk was a major export of the Chinese and the deer was, accordingly, a highly valued animal and a popular subject for artists

Right: a Persian lady with an amphora-shaped vessel intended for scented drinks and sherbets.

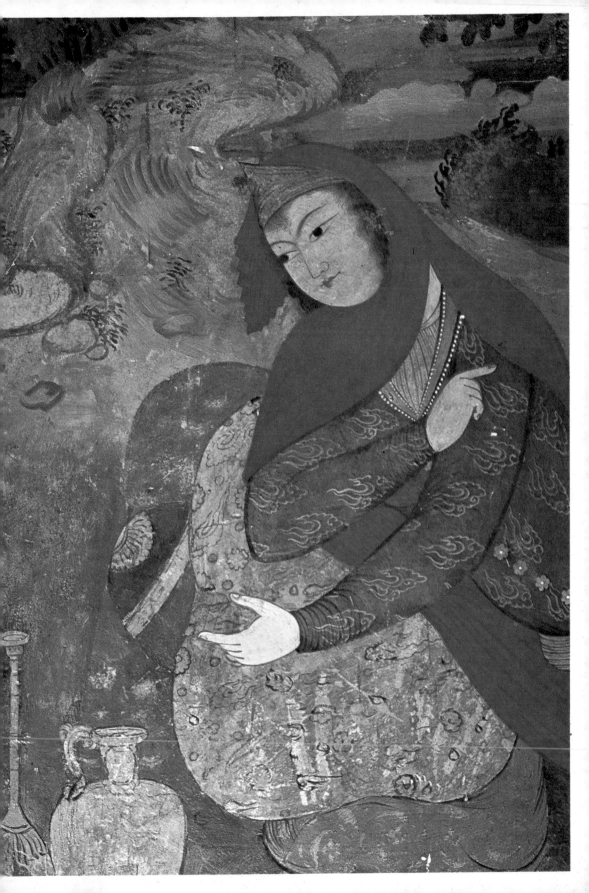

Violet

The scent of the violet is as fleeting and transient as that of musk is long-lasting. Shakespeare described the violet's character as:

Forward, not permanent; sweet, not lasting.
The perfume and suppliance of a minute.

This elusive quality is caused by a substance known as ionine within the violet flower. Ionine has the power quickly to inhibit the sense of smell. So it is not the violet that loses its fragrance; it is we who lose our ability to smell it. If we allow a few minutes for our sense of smell to recover, we shall once again smell the violet. And once again the scent will fade. One of the delights of the violet is thus that it is never possible to be surfeited by its perfume. We can never get enough.

So much in demand was the violet for its perfume that, long before the birth of Christ, it was cultivated commercially in Athens. And so important was it to the Athenians that they made it the symbol of their city. The flowers were used by the Greeks mainly to perfume their wines.

The Greeks can be forgiven for not making a perfume, in our modern usage of the word, from violets. In spite of its botanical name, *Viola odorata,* the violet is one of the most difficult of all flowers in the obstinancy with which it resists attempts to extract its perfume. Violet absolute – the completely pure and unadulterated liquid perfume – is obtained by enfleurage or by the rather similar process of maceration. In enfleurage, as we have already seen, cold fat is used; in maceration the flower petals are soaked in hot fat, which is dissolved away to leave the absolute. Both processes are expensive. Writing in the latter half of the 19th century, Charles Piesse, in his *Art of Perfumery,* tells us that even then 'the demand for the "essence of violets" is far greater than the manufacturing perfumers are able to supply, and, as a consequence, it is difficult to procure the genuine article through the ordinary sources of trade.

'Real violet is, however, sold by many of the retail perfumers of the West End of London, but at a price that prohibits its use except by the affluent or extravagant votaries of fashion.'

The situation is, of course, worse today, and most violet used in modern perfumery is synthetic. Nonetheless, violet absolute, like that of the rose, jasmine, and orange blossom, is still important in the production of expensive perfumes for the luxury market.

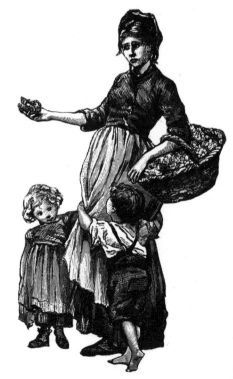

Sweet Violets ! – a street flower-seller in London in the 1880s.

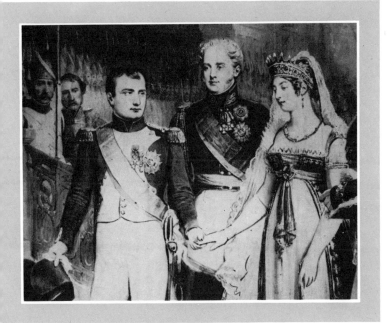

Napoleon and Josephine at Tilsit, 1807. Josephine delighted in the scent of violets and frequently wore a violet perfume. When she died, in 1814, Napoleon had her grave covered with violet plants. Shortly before he went to St. Helena on his final exile he visited Josephine's grave and picked some of the flowers from it. After his death these flowers were found, crushed, in a locket he had always worn around his neck.

A Spode porcelain violet basket of about 1820.

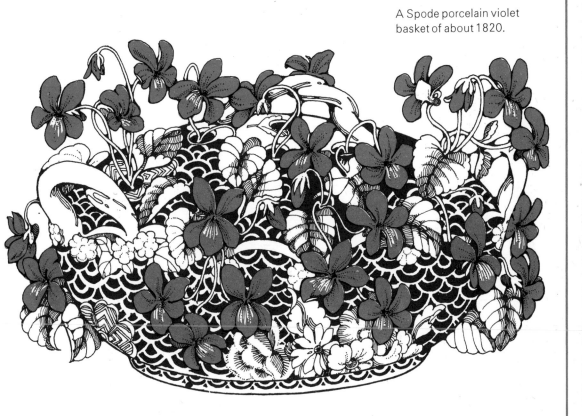

بُوي كُوز بُوي كجُرِي كلِ چنبِيلِي بُوي بِنك تُرنج

بُوي نِيلِه عَنبَر اشهب كلِ چنبِه بُوي كلِ جايِي جُويِي

بُوي بَرك لِمُو بُوي بِدهَل بُوي پُوست كرِنه سلارِس

بُوي بَالا

قَرنَفَل

بُوي

مُوز

كلِ تُرنج

بُوي صَمدَك دِيكَر انواع دَتهَارَه دَتهَارَه رُوهَس

دَتهَارَه اسِير دَتهَارَه بَالا دَتهَارَه تُلسِي وازبَرَك تخان

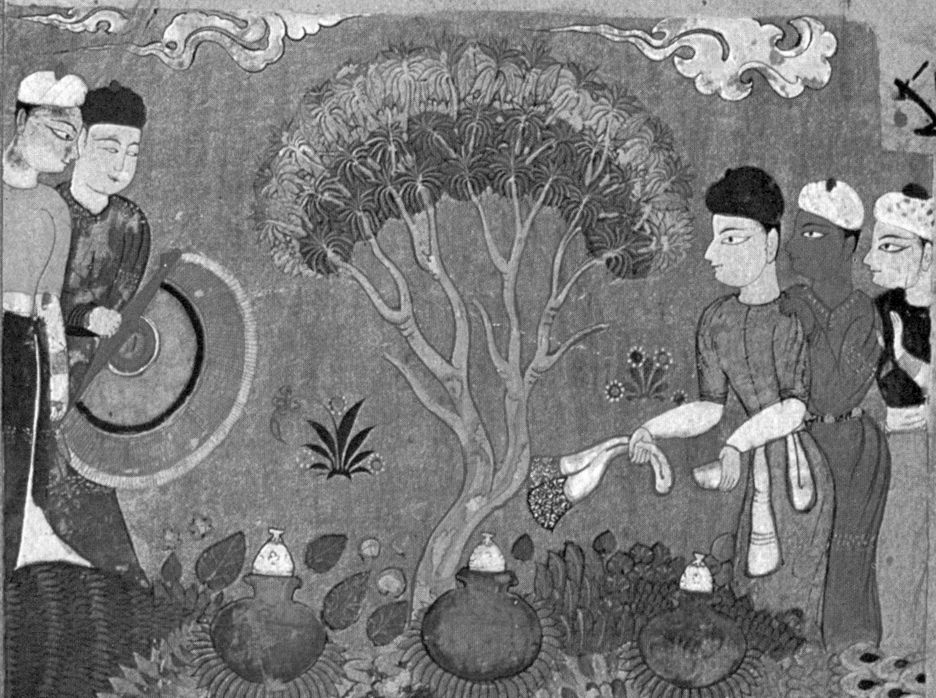

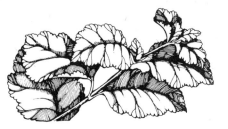

Patchouli

Patchouli is a scent obtained from the leaves and stems of the herb *Pogostemon patchouli,* a member of the lavender family and a native of Bengal. Attar of patchouli is obtained from the plant by distillation; one hundredweight of leaves and stems produces about 30 ounces of the dark brown, oily attar.

Patchouli is the most powerful of all the scents obtained from plants. In its unadulterated state it is, in the words of the 19th-century perfumer Charles Piesse, 'far from agreeable, having a kind of mossy or musty odour . . . it smells of "old coats".' Not surprisingly, it is normally used heavily diluted and in small quantities.

It is patchouli, plus camphor, that gives Indian ink its characteristic smell. In the East, dried crushed leaves of patchouli are commonly used for scenting linen – they are supposed to have moth-repellent qualities. In the West, attar of patchouli is used in the manufacture of some hair oils and shampoos.

Patchouli came to Europe by an odd route. There was in Victorian times a craze for cashmere shawls – the queen herself is wearing one in the photograph (*right*). British manufacturers tried to cash in on the fashion by making imitation shawls – machine-made, they could be produced more cheaply than the originals. But Indian shawls were easily distinguishable from the imitations because a whiff of patchouli always clung to them. So British manufacturers began to import patchouli to scent their home-produced shawls. Perfumers then discovered the scent and began to market *Extract of Patchouli,* which was attar of patchouli mixed with attar of roses and heavily diluted with spirits of wine.

Left: page from an Indian 'cookery book' of about 1500. The manuscript shows a method of perfuming water, using the various flowers and leaves described in the text.

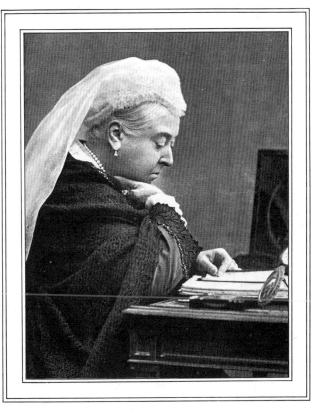

Vetivert

Vetivert is extracted from the roots of a grass, *Vetiveria zizanioides,* which grows in India, Burma, and Sri Lanka, on the island of Réunion in the West Indies, and in Central and South America. Essence of vetivert, which was fashionable in Georgian and early Victorian times among the wives of retired Indian merchants and officials, was made by steeping the dried, powdered roots in spirits of wine.

Vetivert was the basis of another 19th-century perfume, *Mousseline des Indes.* This took its name from India muslin, which used to be scented with vetivert, to make it moth- and insect-proof, before being exported to Europe. Two other Victorian perfumes, *Maréchale* and *Bouquet de Roi,* were also based on vetivert.

It is not a popular scent today, although it is still used to some extent in shampoos and in face creams and lipsticks. Its main value to the modern perfumer is as a fixative and as such it is to be found in several manufactured perfumes.

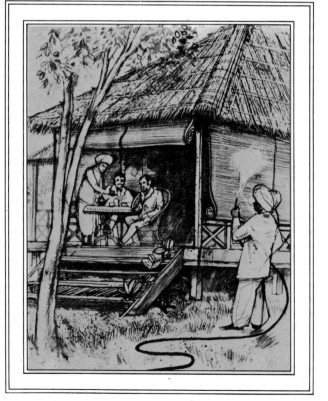

In the time of the Georgian dandy (*right*), men as well as women used essence of vetivert, particularly as a handkerchief perfume. It was a reminder at home of Britain's Indian possessions. In India itself the root of vetivert is traditionally woven into screens or awnings called *tatties.* Hung over doors and windows, or used as wall hangings, they are sprinkled with water (*left*), so that evaporation cools the room and at the same time scents it with a violet-like perfume. Some of the vetivert that found its way on to the European market was root that had been used in *tatties* for a season and reclaimed for sale to the perfumer after it had been largely exhausted of its oils by constant exposure to the sun.

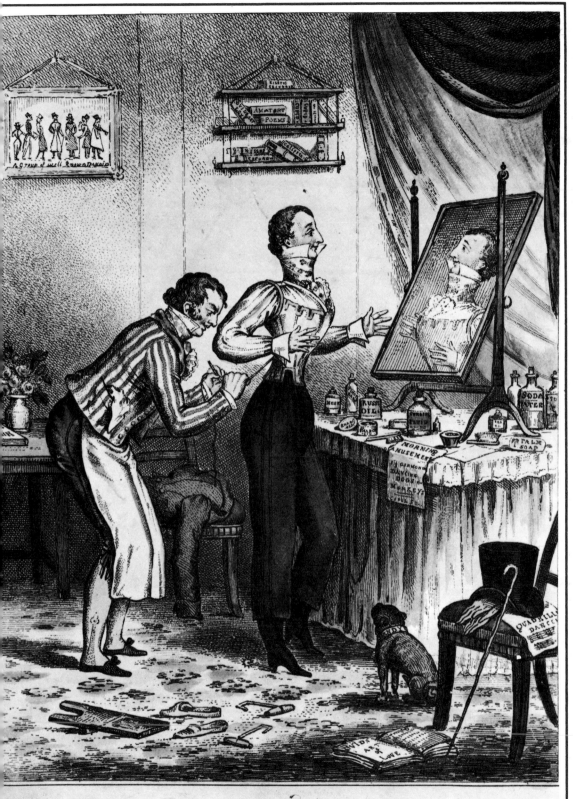

DANDY'S TOILETTE.
Stays;

Cedarwood

Cedarwood yields an essential oil which gives – naturally enough – a woody undertone to a perfume and which is valuable as a fixative. Tincture of cedar can be made simply by steeping chips of the wood in proof spirit. Cedarwood sawdust can be used as an ingredient of pot-pourris. But cedarwood is not particularly important to the modern perfumer. It was used to a rather greater extent in the 19th century. Cedarwood matches enjoyed a brief popularity, and little slabs of cedarwood were sometimes put into drawers among the linen to discourage moths. Attar of cedar was an ingredient of 'cold cream soap' and, diluted with spirits of wine, was used to saturate handkerchiefs. One Victorian perfumer bought waste cedar from a pencil manufacturer to make 'Lebanon Cedar Wood for the handkerchief'. (There was at the time no Trade Descriptions Act. Had there been, someone might have pointed out that the pencil wood was American cedar, *Juniperus virginiana,* not the Lebanon cedar, *Cedrus Libani.*) None of this comes anywhere near the extensive use of cedar that was made in ancient times. Ground cedar was used by the Egyptians in the making of incense. Oil of cedarwood was used in the mummification process and was also used to smear over papyrus leaves to protect them from insect attack.

Today the best cedarwood for the perfumer comes from trees grown in the Atlas Mountains of Morocco. But the trees that figure most prominently in the history of perfumery are the cedars of Lebanon. Few of these remain. The mountains of Lebanon were once densely covered with a prolific growth of immense cedar trees, but wholesale felling reduced the forests to scattered groups of trees even in ancient times. By the time of Alexander the Great, the apparently inexhaustible forests of Lebanon were no more. At the beginning of our own century it was recorded that 'Of the chief ornament of Lebanon in ancient time, the cedars, there still exist small groups in many places . . . the largest consisting of about 350 trees . . . .' In recent years there have been attempts at reafforestation, but none of these have been very successful. The shoots of the young trees have proved irresistible to mountain goats.

The cedar forests of Lebanon were wiped out by the demands made upon them by the builders of antiquity. Cedarwood was a building material employed in all the great temples and palaces of the Middle East. One violater of the forests was King Solomon, who imported vast quantities of cedar to build his great temple in Jerusalem. The temple – the first of three built on the same site – stood for almost 400 years; it was demolished by Nebuchadnezzar in about 586 B.C. *Right,* the massive cedars for Solomon's temple begin their journey to Jerusalem.

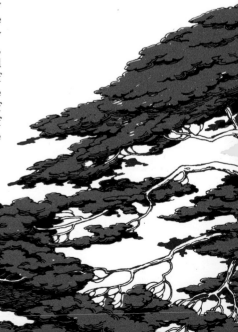

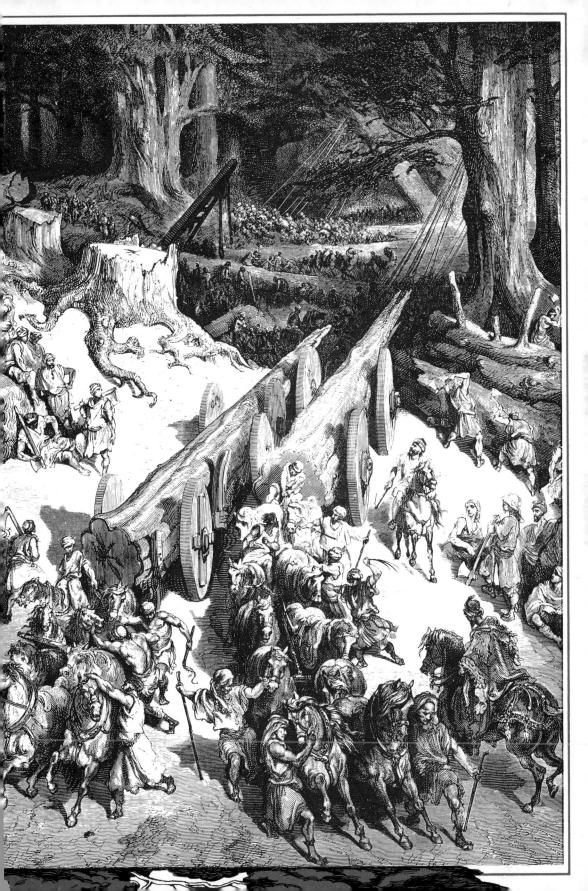

Cedarwood was in very great demand in the ancient world not only because of the aesthetic appeal of its scent. It was valued for practical reasons. Like sandalwood, it was hard enough to resist attack by woodboring insects and its scent also was thought to be insect-repellent. It was therefore much used in the building of temples and palaces, whose gates and roof-beams were almost always made of cedar.

The biggest buyers and users were Egypt and Mesopotamia, both of which lacked home-grown timber. The Phoenicians who controlled the cedar forests found themselves sitting on a fortune. The difficulty was getting the massive trunks of cedar to their destinations. They were hauled down from the mountains by teams of oxen, dragged across the Aleppo plain, and, if destined for Mesopotamia, floated down the Euphrates. The amount of labour involved was immense.

It was the export of cedar to Egypt that was the most profitable. The Egyptians ate up cedar. They needed it not only for their buildings but also for their ships. For the Mediterranean coastal trade, and for local journeys on the Nile, the Egyptians found papyrus boats adequate. But the Red Sea could be dangerous; it demanded the strong cedarwood ships in whose construction the Phoenicians had a near-monopoly. So the Phoenicians had it both ways – they were both the manufacturers and the suppliers of raw materials to the Egyptian pharaohs. The massive trunks of cedar were carried to the Lebanese coast and shipped – on Phoenician vessels – to Egypt's north coast. There they were off-loaded and taken overland to one of the Egyptian ports on the Red Sea, where Phoenician shipwrights were waiting. The Egyptians never mastered the skills of shipbuilding. They relied on the expertise of the Phoenicians, who built for them ships that then often sailed with combined Phoenician-Egyptian crews.

These, of course, were merchant ships, many of them engaged in the incense trade. But cedarwood was also used in the construction of the ceremonial boats that were so dear to the hearts of the Egyptian pharaohs. Cleopatra's barge was one of a long line. Every pharaoh had to have his own barge. Lavishly gilded, splendidly equipped, sometimes 200 feet long, they were the most breathtakingly magnificent state barges of all time.

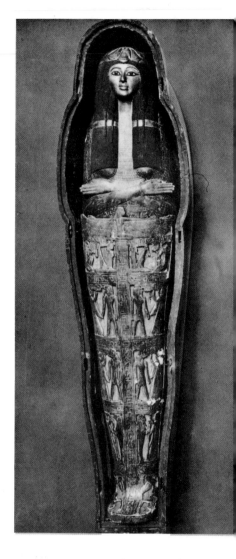

Above: the mummy cover and coffin of Henutmehit, a priestess of Amun, who died in about 1300 B.C. Cedarwood, because it was both durable and pleasantly scented, was always the material preferred by Egyptian coffin-makers for expensive coffins such as this. Many of them survive today – still in good condition after 3,000 years.

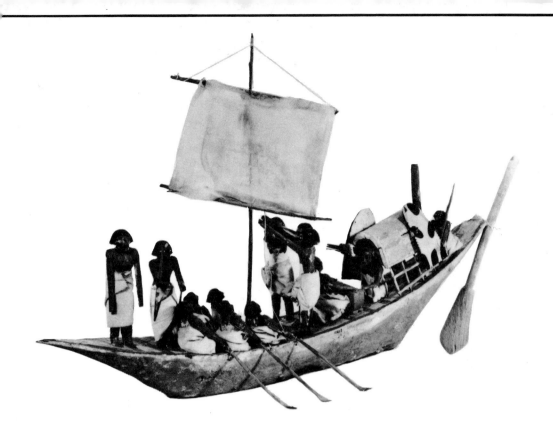

Above: a wooden model of an Egyptian boat of about 1900 B.C. Although this one is carrying soldiers, it is probably very like the cedarwood ships built by Phoenician shipwrights for the Egyptian merchant fleets. The typical merchant ship of this period was some 70 feet long overall; it carried its cargo on its single deck.

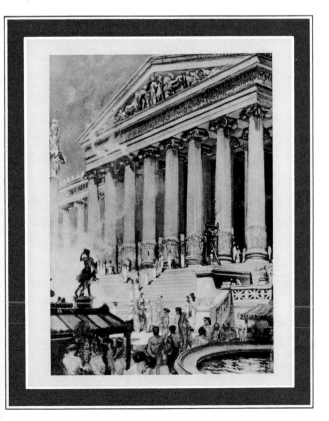

Left: another famous building in whose construction cedarwood was used – the temple of Diana at Ephesus, built in the 6th century B.C. and burned to the ground, so legend has it, in 356 B.C., on the night Alexander the Great was born. The huge temple was one of the Seven Wonders of the ancient world. It covered over an acre of ground and its columns were 55 feet high and 6 feet thick at the base.

Clove

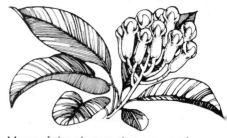

The cloves that we find in apple pies are the un-expanded flower buds of the clove tree *Caryophyllus aromaticus*. The same buds provide the perfumer with his attar of cloves. Cloves are best known as a spice. Through ancient and medieval times, before ways of preserving meats were found, they were an important and valuable article of commerce, being imported into Europe from the Far East. They have, however, a respectable history in perfumery. Centuries before Christ, envoys to the Han court of China held cloves in their mouths to freshen their breath during audiences with the emperor. In the 19th century A.D. cloves were frequently the main ingredient of handkerchief essences, including one with the high-camp name of *The Guards' Bouquet*.

Today Zanzibar has a near-monopoly of the production of cloves. In the Middle Ages, the world's supplies all came from Indonesia and the East Indies. Then, in the second half of the 18th century, the French began growing cloves in Mauritius and from there they were quickly introduced into Zanzibar. In 1974 the crop – from which the island gets 90 per cent of its income – was hit by a disease that turned the trees grey and stunted the growth of the all-important flower buds.

Many of the plagues that scourged Europe were started by fleas carried by rats that came ashore from ships bringing spices from the East. So cloves have a share in the responsibility for plagues. With poetic justice, they were also used as a prophylactic against bubonic plague. Sponges impregnated with extract of cloves were often held beneath the noses of plague victims. The 17th-century plague doctor (*right*) is wearing the protective clothing of his profession – a leather gown, leather gloves, and a leather mask. The beak through which he breathes is filled with cloves, cinnamon, and other spices and aromatics. He carries a wand so that he does not have to touch his patients with his hands – he even felt their pulses with it. There is some modern evidence that suggests that cloves might have had some real medical value; one researcher has reported that oil of cloves kills the bacillus that causes typhoid.

Right: an Arab dhow engaged in the export trade in cloves from Zanzibar a hundred years ago. Zanzibar today supplies the world. It even supplies Indonesia, the original home of cloves. This is because the Dutch, to discourage the Indonesians from chewing betel nuts, tried in the late 19th century to convert them to cigarette smoking. They introduced cigarettes made from the local tobacco and ground cloves, mixed in the proportion of 2 to 1. These cigarettes caught on to such an extent that for their manufacture Indonesia has to import from Zanzibar 6,000 tons of cloves a year.

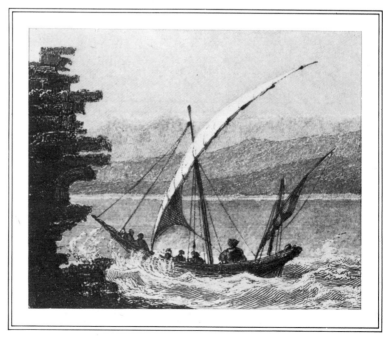

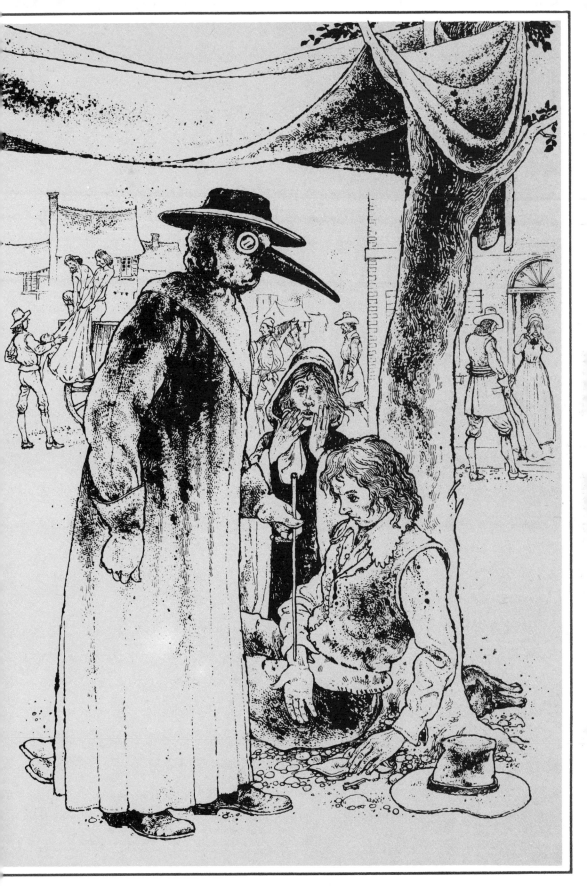

Castoreum

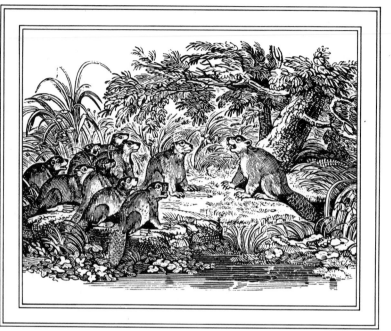

Castoreum is beaver oil. Like ambergris, civet, and musk it is an animal product used by the perfumer as a fixative and as a blender. In its dry state – it comes in brittle pear-shaped sacs like half-deflated balloons – castoreum has very little smell. Its odour develops when it is dissolved in spirits of wine. It is then potent and overpowering – so much so that if mixed with other scents in any proportion greater than about 1 in 40 its odour totally overwhelms the others. It is not now very popular with the commercial perfume manufacturers, partly because supplies are short and prices are high, partly because it has become unfashionable, and partly because it does nothing that musk, civet, or a synthetic cannot do better. Even that dedicated perfumer Charles Piesse, writing in 1891, was scornful of castoreum. He used it in none of his perfume recipes and dismissed it in a scathing sentence: 'Perfumes containing it last well on the handkerchief, but there are very few persons who consider it nice.' In Piesse's day, castoreum was imported from Canada and was a monopoly of the Hudson's Bay Company.

Left: a colony of beavers, from Simeon Shaw's *Nature Displayed,* published in 1823. *Right:* a 19th-century engraving of a beaver doing what is expected of it – felling a tree to make a dam. Castoreum comes from the groin of the Canadian and Siberian beaver; the sacs in which it arrives at the perfumer's warehouse are in fact dried lymphatic glands. Supplies of castoreum tend to be seasonal. This is because the beaver is killed for its fur; castoreum is only a by-product. Most beavers are trapped in winter, when their fur is at its best and when they assemble in colonies so that they are easier to hunt than in the summer, when they live in isolated pairs.

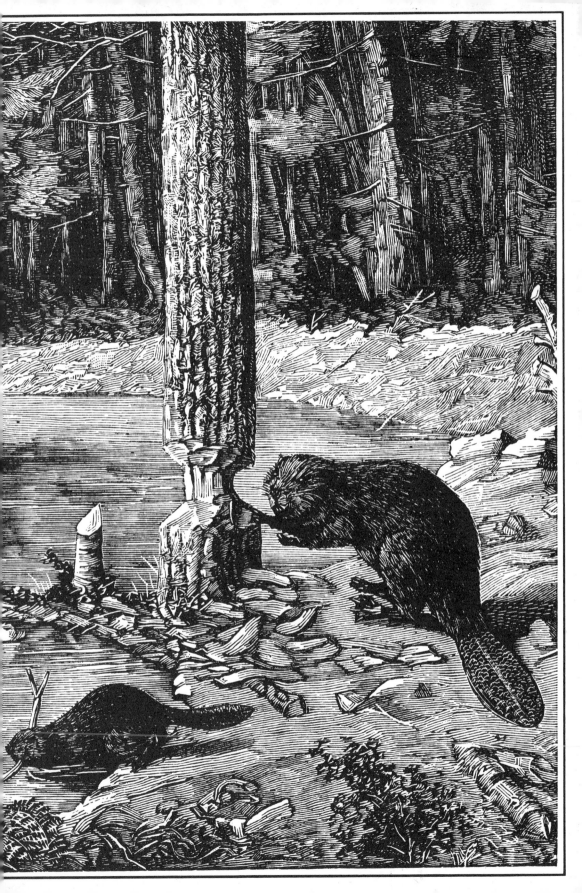

Ambergris

Ambergris is the most legendary of all perfume materials. Its origins and nature were long unknown. Thousands of years ago fishermen and sailors first found mysterious, oily, ash-grey lumps floating on the surface of the warm seas. They thought it to be some sort of vegetable matter and called it 'grey amber'. Over the centuries a variety of theories to explain it were put forward. A certain M. de Moncomys reported in 1725 that he had been told – 'in England' – that 'ambergris was nothing but honeycombs that bees make upon the large rocks, which are on the Sea Side in the Indies, which, heated by the Sun, loosen and fall into the Sea'. Sindbad the Sailor, whose fabulous voyages are related in the *Arabian Nights' Entertainments,* had his own explanation. Somewhere on the Indian coast, he says, 'is a fountain of pitch and bitumen, that runs into the sea, which the fishes swallow, and then vomit it up again, turned into ambergris'. Sindbad had come quite close to the truth, although he was wrong about both the bitumen and the fish. Ambergris is formed by a mammal – the sperm whale – in an odd way. The whale's diet includes whole squids and cuttlefish and parts of these fish, in particular the 'beak' of the cuttlefish, are difficult for the whale's digestive juices to cope with. Some whales – perhaps sickly ones – manage to protect their stomachs by thickly coating the indigestible lumps with a kind of wax. The coated lumps are eventually excreted by the whale and float to the surface of the sea.

Now that intensive whaling has almost wiped out the sperm whale, ambergris is likely to become even rarer and even costlier and, eventually, to disappear completely from the seas. Chemists have, however, recently succeeded in producing a synthetic substitute.

In spite of its unlikely origins, ambergris is one of the ingredients perfumers use to give sexiness to a scent. They use it, of course, heavily diluted. (It dissolves in alcohol, although not in water.) In its concentrated state it is, in Rimmel's phrase, 'not agreeable by itself'. The smell of crude ambergris was trenchantly, if indirectly, described by Wilhelm Homberg, the German chemist who discovered boracic acid, in 1711: '. . . a vessel in which I had made a long digestion of human faeces had acquired a very strong and perfect smell of ambergris, insomuch that anyone would have thought that a great quantity of essence of ambergris had been made in it . . . the perfume was so strong that the vessel was obliged to be moved out of the laboratory.'

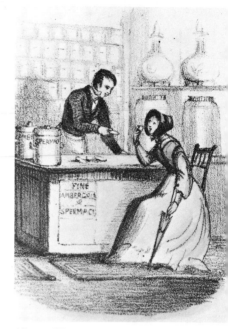

Above: 'Fine Ambergris and Spermaceti.' Both the wares advertised by this retailer were products of the whaling industry. Spermaceti, a waxy solid obtained from whale oil, was used in soaps, ointments, and candles.

Far right: a whaler meets disaster off the coast of Greenland. Until the 18th century the only whales killed by men were those that became stranded or strayed too close to the shore. Then whaling was organized into an industry and fleets of ships began to make long voyages to hunt down whales. The Dutch, who dominated the whaling industry, started to cut up the whales for their blubber on board ship and found pieces of ambergris in the stomachs. They were the first to connect ambergris with the whale. But most ambergris continued to come from pieces found floating on the sea. The largest single haul of ambergris pieces was collected in 1880 by a Dutch East Indiaman which landed about nine hundredweight. The biggest single piece ever found was a lump 60 inches long by about 30 inches in diameter, weighing over three hundredweight, that was discovered in 1953. Ambergris is usually found in far smaller pieces, weighing about a pound and worth at today's prices well over £100.

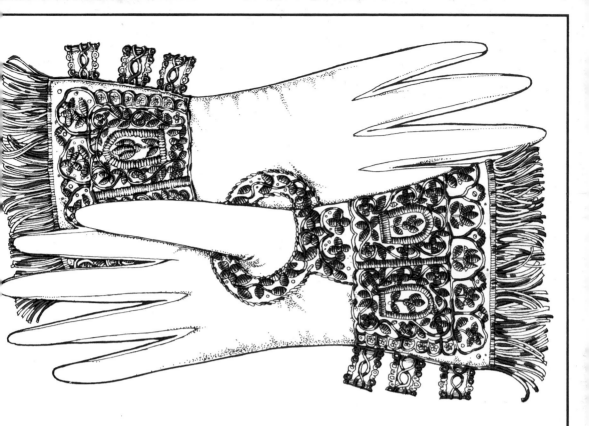

Ambergris was often used to perfume gloves, such as those that Elizabeth I was fond of wearing (*above*). It had the advantage of retaining its scent after repeated washings. Elizabeth wore, on special occasions, a cloak made of perfumed leather and also had several pairs of shoes of the same material. The probability is that these too were scented with ambergris,

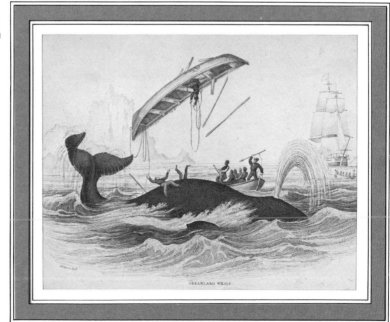

GREENLAND WHALE

Civet

Civet, which often scented the more elaborate of Victorian valentines, is another romantic scent of unromantic origin. It comes from a wild and un-endearing animal, the civet cat. It is the secretion from a gland situated underneath the civet's tail. In its raw state – it is an unattractive yellowish-brown substance – it smells disgusting. Heavily diluted, and mixed with other scents, it becomes attractive. Diluted, however, it must be, otherwise it is repellent rather than seductive. In the early 17th century, when civet was passing through one of its phases as a fashionable glove scent, the dramatist Philip Massinger spelled out the danger:

Lady, I would descend to kiss thy hand,

But that 'tis gloved, and civet makes me sick.

Charles Piesse, although committed to civet's attraction, advised care in its use. 'The odour of civet', he wrote, 'is best imparted, not by actual contact, but by being placed in the neighbourhood of absorbent materials. Thus, when spread upon leather, and placed in a writing-desk, it perfumes the paper and envelopes delightfully, so much so that they retain the odour after passing through the post.' Nonetheless, discreetly used, civet is invaluable as a fixative; it is fonud in surprisingly many modern perfumes.

Right: the frontispiece of *Parfumeur Françoys,* published in Paris in 1680, shows some of the sources of the substances then used in perfumery. In the foreground are two civets, one caged and one being killed — unnecessarily — for its scent sac. Behind them is a man combing the beard of a mountain goat to collect myrrh. It is still the practice today, as it was in Solomon's time, to gather myrrh gum-resin by sending goats into the inaccessible places where the prickly myrrh shrub grows. The goats nibble at the bark and collect the sticky gum on their beards. The potted plants in the picture are probably orange trees. Floating on the sea is an improbable islet made up of pieces of ambergris.

Right: the civet cat lives, in the wild, in Malaysia, Java, Sri Lanka, India, and Africa. Most of the civet used in perfumery comes from animals kept in captivity in Africa. The Dutch seem to have been the first to have kept civets for this purpose on an industrial scale — a number were brought to Amsterdam in the 19th century. The cats were put into wooden cages so narrow that they could not turn round. The contents of the scent gland could then be removed, in safety, with a small spoon. The cats were said to produce larger quantities of civet when they were bad-tempered.

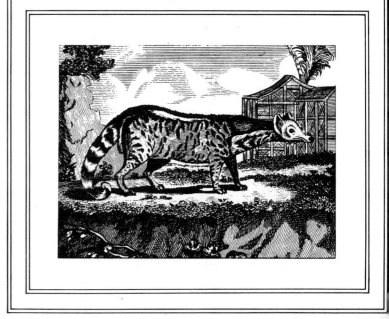

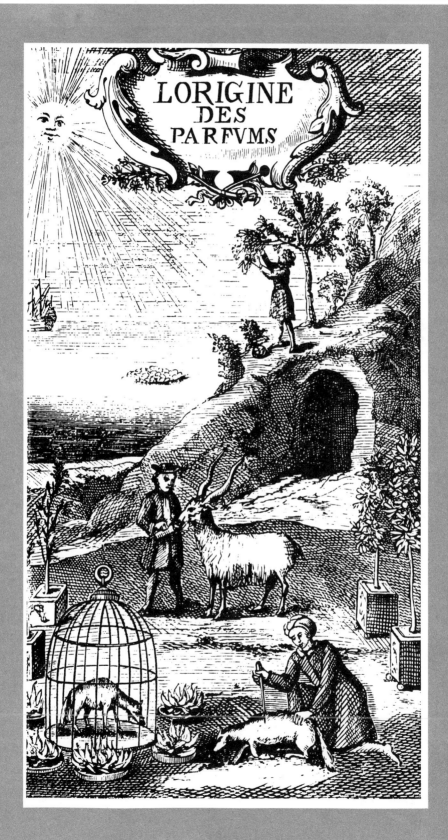

LORIGINE
DES
PARFVMS

Lavender

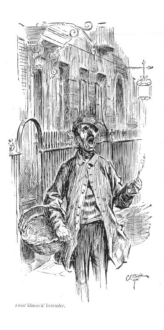

Sweet bloomin' lavender.

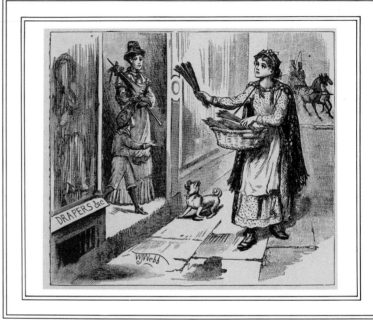

Our word 'lavender' comes from the Latin *lavare*, to wash. The derivation is appropriate – lavender is, in Rimmel's gentle words, 'a nice, *clean* scent, and an old and deserving favourite'. The Romans steeped the leaves and stems of the lavender plant in the water they used for their baths and thus began the association of lavender with freshness that has lasted to this day. They probably introduced the plant into Britain, where it was grown in cottage gardens as long as there were cottage gardens to grow it in.

Roman lavender water was simply an infusion of lavender in water. Later, lavender water was obtained from the plant by distillation. In the 16th century lavender water was distilled in many English country houses and by the 17th century the home distillation of lavender became as popular a hobby as home wine-making is today. Leisured women gave over whole rooms to lavender distilling and invited their friends in for lavender-smelling sessions.

Today's best-known lavender water – Yardley's – is more complicated than the water these ladies made. It is based upon oil of lavender – obtained by distillation – but contains many other ingredients, including attar of roses, French rose absolute, musk, and neroli.

Above: 'Buy my sweet lavender, two bunches a penny' was one of the street cries of old London. In 1913 the firm of Yardley borrowed an engraving from the 'Cries of London' series by Francis Wheatley to advertise their *Old English Lavender.* Unable to find a lavender seller, Yardley's made do with a primrose seller, touching out her primroses and replacing them with lavender.

Below: lavender pickers in the south of France, where the plants still have to be hand-cut with sickles. Lavender is a major crop of French Alpine farmers, who produce most of the lavender for commercial use. The blossoms are harvested in July and August each year. In Britain, Mitcham in Surrey was the first and biggest centre for lavender growing, but lavender was also cultivated and distilled in Hertfordshire, in Lincolnshire, and in Norfolk — the county that still provides some of the lavender for Yardley. The British harvest is about a month later than the French. The best known of commercial lavenders is Yardley's, whose *English Lavender* is something stronger than a toilet water yet less concentrated than a perfume. (The difference between perfume and toilet water is mainly that of dilution — perfume has a greater proportion of pure fragrance mixed with its alcohol base.) Yardley's came into the perfume business early in the 19th century when William Yardley, a Bloomsbury sword-cutler, foreclosed on the failed soap and perfumery business of his son-in-law William Cleaver. Cleaver's company had been founded in 1770 and was probably using lavender from the beginning. Men were starting to go wigless and, to display their hair to best advantage, used hair grease and hair oils in great quantity. A hair dressing of bear's grease scented with lavender became a best seller. The new firm of Yardley became in time the world's largest manufacturer of lavender products.

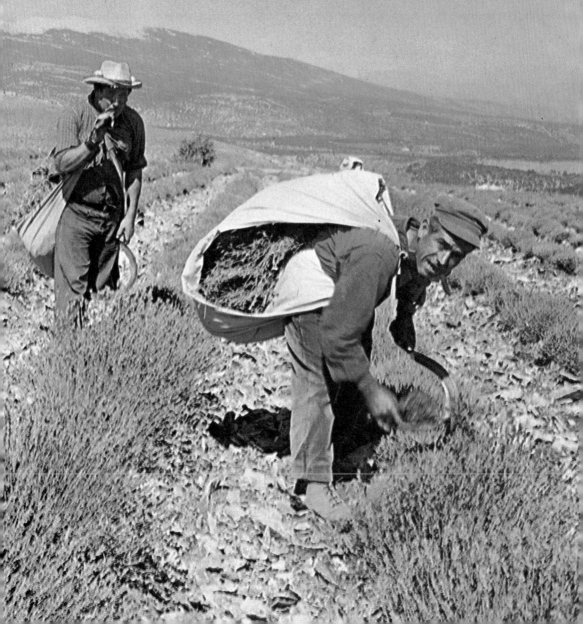

Lemon Grass

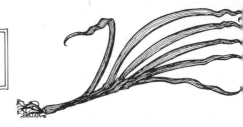

Lemon grass has nothing to do with the lemon, nor is it a single grass. The oil used in perfumery is, properly, that distilled from *Andropogon citratus,* a species of grass native to the Indian sub-continent. Nineteenth-century perfumers got their supplies from Ceylon and the Moluccas. It was imported from there into Britain, for some extraordinary but unfathomable reason, in second-hand stout and porter bottles. The attar was in those days cheap and strong and hence popular with the perfumer. Other related grasses also produce lemon-grass attar. *Cymbopogon nardus* grows widely in the Middle East. *Cymbopogon schöenanthus* grows in Egypt and Arabia and has a subtle rose-like scent; it is sometimes used to adulterate attar of roses. It was one of the ingredients of the holy anointing oil with which Aaron and his sons were consecrated. Nowadays it may occasionally appear disguised as 'oil of geranium'. *Andropogon nardus,* native to India and Sri Lanka, is used to give a 'honey' scent to soaps.

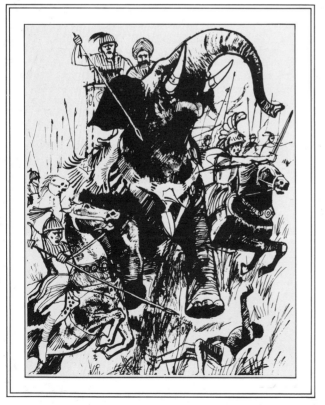

Left: the story goes that Alexander the Great, riding on an elephant near the borders of Egypt, suddenly smelled spikenard and was intoxicated by the scent. It is much more probable that what Alexander smelled was the grass *Cymbopogon nardus,* whose scent – given off when the grass is crushed by a human foot, much less an elephant's – is very much like that of spikenard. Alexander entered Egypt – then a Persian province – in 332 B.C. The country surrendered to him without a struggle; he entered Memphis more as a liberator than a conqueror and was hailed as pharaoh. Early in 331, he went to consult the oracle of Amun (*right*) at the Siwa oasis on the other side of the Libyan desert. The oracle, recognizing *force majeure* when he saw it, declared Alexander to be the divine son of the god Amun and so gave theological respectability to Alexander's rule.

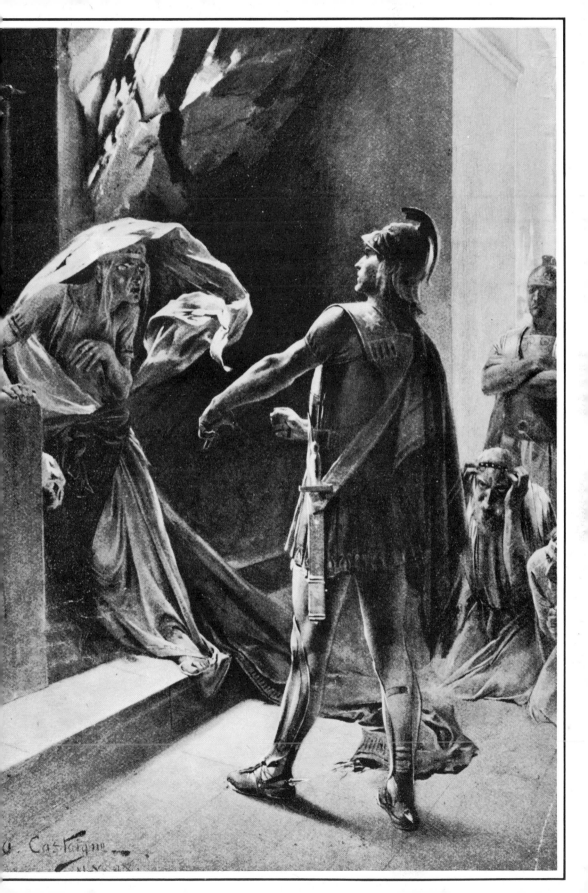

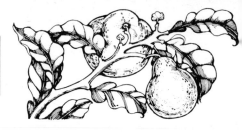

Neroli

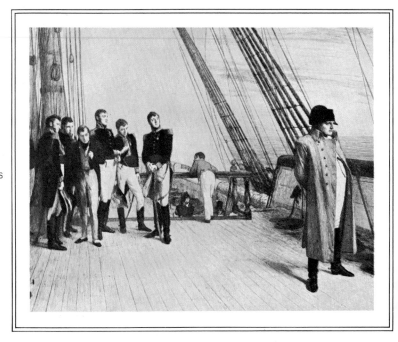

Right: Napoleon on board the 'Bellerophon', the ship that took him to exile on St. Helena after his defeat at Waterloo — from the familiar painting by Sir William Orchardson. Napoleon's final exile took him permanently from Paris and parted him from his perfumer 'by appointment', Chardin. Napoleon had for many years had a standing order with Chardin for eau de Cologne. In one quarter of 1806, 162 bottles were delivered to him; in one quarter of 1810, 144 bottles. Later, Chardin supplied the emperor with 648 bottles of an 'improved' quality — probably a more concentrated cologne.

Neroli oil is distilled from the bloom of the bitter orange tree, *Citrus bigaradia,* the only tree whose flowers, leaves, and fruit all yield materials for the perfumer. Why attar of oranges should be called neroli is something of a mystery. It has been suggested, rather implausibly, that the scent took its name from that great perfume-lover, the emperor Nero. Piesse suggests that the word is even earlier: 'it may be that "Neroli" was first procured by the Sabines, who, to distinguish it from other perfumes of the period, named it neroli, from "nero", which signifies "strong".' The currently accepted story is that neroli gets its name from a prince of Nerola, Flavio Orsini, member of a famous Roman family, who lived in the 16th century and whose wife scented her bath and her gloves with the perfume. This fits rather better with the tradition that the orange tree was introduced into Europe only in the 12th century, brought back from the East Indies by Portuguese sailors. Today, neroli oil comes from the south of France, Morocco, Tunisia, Sicily, and the United States of America. Neroli is an important ingredient in many modern perfumes, including, surprisingly, lavender water.

Neroli oil is, and always has been, a basic constituent of eau de Cologne, which is a concoction of neroli and other orange attars, mixed with rosemary and bergamot and dissolved in spirits of wine. Bergamot, like neroli, is an orange product; it is extracted from the rind of the pear-shaped orange *Citrus bergamia.* In Napoleon's time bergamot was produced in Lombardy: today most supplies come from Calabria, in the toe of Italy. It is used especially in after-shave lotions, such as Yardley's *Black Label.* Bergamot is one of the clean, 'fresh' scents, like lavender; it smells very much like the rosemary with which it is mixed in eau de Cologne. It was perhaps the rosemary scent of eau de Cologne that appealed to Napoleon.; it may have reminded him of his boyhood in Corsica (*right*), where rosemary grew wild in the thick, scrubby underbrush of the *maquis.*

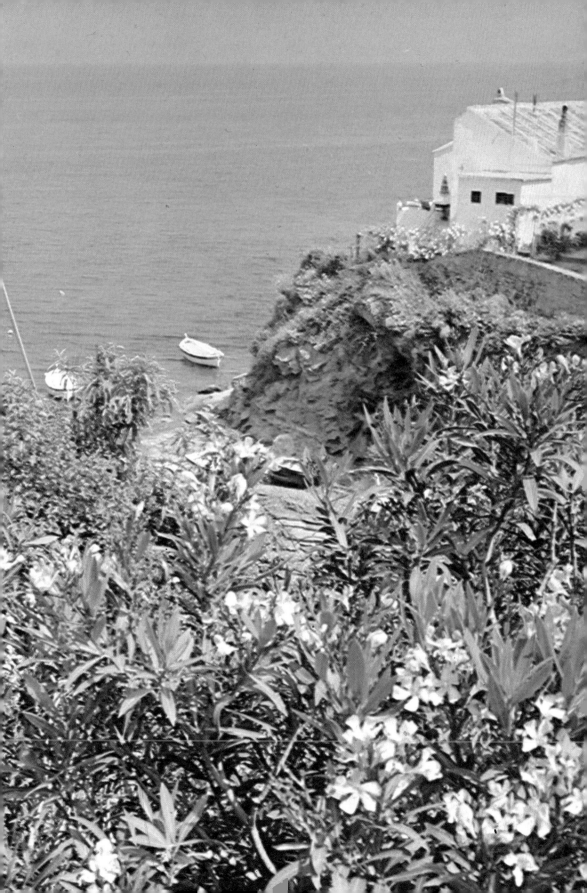

Frankincense

Frankincense is a fragrant gum exuded by the shrubby trees *Boswellia carterii* and *Boswellia serrata* – both of which are related to the terebinth tree – which grew on the southern coasts of Arabia and in east Africa. As the trees grow only on rocky hillsides and in steep ravines, collecting the gum has always presented difficulties. Together with myrrh – with which its history is almost inextricably interwoven – frankincense was one of the most highly prized substances of the ancient world. It was the gum most frequently burned as incense – so much so that 'incense' is often used simply as a shorthand term for frankincense.

In the ancient world, frankincense and myrrh were as important in international commerce as is oil today. Because of this they inevitably became factors in international politics. The countries of the Middle East were continually in conflict over control of the sources of supply of incense and of the trade routes along which it was carried. At one time, for example, the south Arabians had to pay an annual tribute – in our terms, protection money – in frankincense to the Persian king Darius to prevent him from taking over the incense-growing region of their land.

The land of frankincense was the land of Punt, the area from which the ancient Egyptians obtained the incense they burned in vast quantities in their temples. No one quite knows where Punt was. The best guess is that it straddled the Red Sea – we know that it possessed territory in both Asia and Africa – at its southern entrance, the strait of Bab el Mandeb. In other words it sounds very much as though Punt was another, perhaps earlier, name for the legendary kingdom of Sheba. The first expedition made by the Egyptians to bring back frankincense from Punt was in the middle of the third millennium B.C. The last was in the reign of the pharaoh Ramses III in the 12th century B.C.

Frankincense was above all a holy perfume. It featured in the religious rites of all the nations of antiquity, especially those of the Israelites. The laws that the Lord gave to Moses were explicit and detailed: 'And thou shalt make an altar to burn incense upon . . . And thou shalt overlay it with pure gold . . . And Aaron shall burn thereon sweet incense every morning: when he dresseth the lamps, he shall burn incense upon it. And . . . at even, he shall burn incense upon it . . . .'

The most extraordinary of the Egyptian expeditions to Punt was undertaken during the reign of Queen Hatshepsut in the 15th century B.C. Egypt at the time was having a balance of payments problem, and Hatshepsut decided that it should grow its own frankincense to cut down on its import bill. To do that she had to buy frankincense trees, from Punt, the only possible supplier. Five ships, like those *below*, set out under the command of Hatshepsut's treasurer and reached Punt after an uneventful voyage. There they were met by the queen of Punt and her daughter, both of whom were grotesquely fat. The treasurer bartered, successfully. The Egyptians loaded their ships (*right*) with frankincense trees, complete with roots and soil, like container-grown plants from a garden centre. Unfortunately, when they got home and planted them in Thebes, the trees refused to grow. The fat queen of Punt had probably seen to it that they wouldn't.

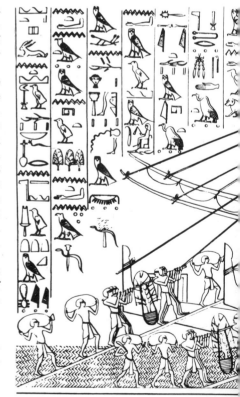

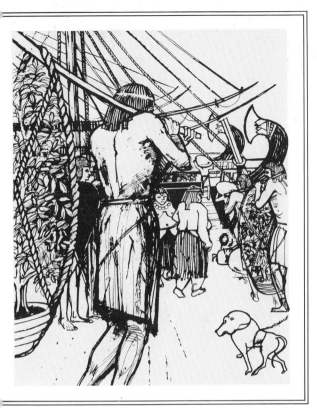

Overleaf: Albrecht Dürer's painting *The Adoration of the Magi* (1504). The three 'wise men' who, according to St Matthew's gospel, came from the East to Jerusalem to do homage to the infant Jesus, bore gifts of gold, frankincense, and myrrh — the three most precious commodities of the age. This, the most famous perfume reference of all time, is the best remembered of all the many biblical allusions to frankincense. It was certainly publicly remembered and celebrated in Britain. When Edward the Confessor founded Westminster Abbey in London in the 11th century, he gave the new church a holy relic — nothing less then some of the frankincense offered by the magi to Jesus. Later English monarchs, up to the time of George III, presented to the chapel of St. James on every Twelfth Night 'three purses filled with gold, frankincense, and myrrh, in commemoration of the presents offered by the Magi'.

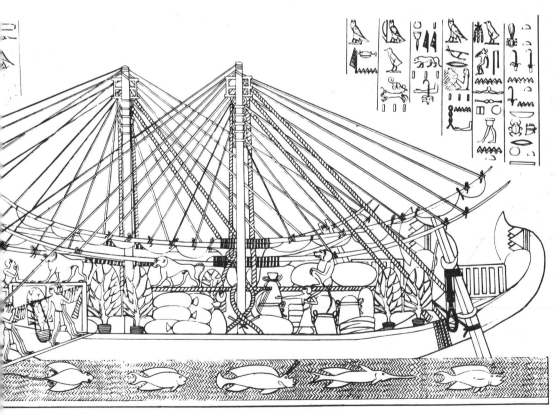

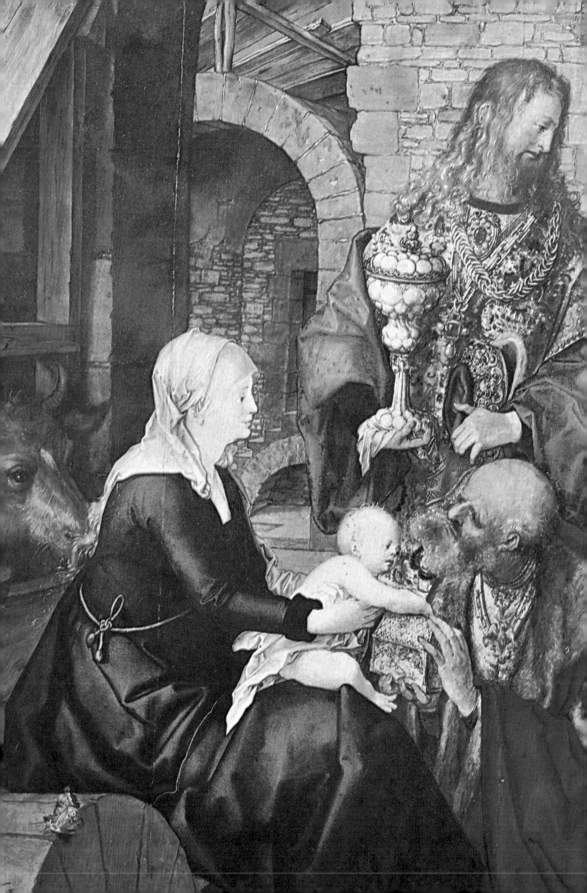

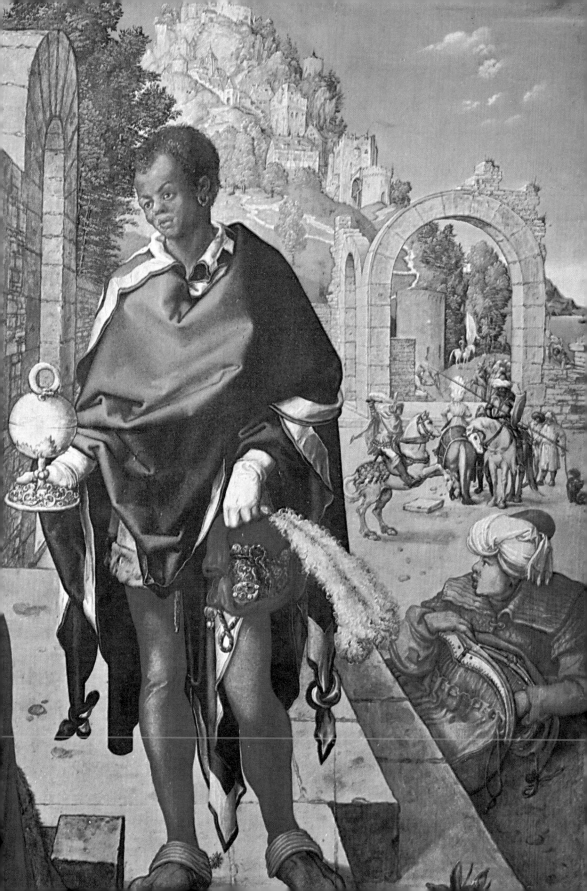

Rose

The most valuable and useful of the natural perfume oils are what are known as 'absolutes'. These are the essential oils extracted from certain flowers – especially the rose, the jasmine, and the violet. Every quality perfume contains a percentage of one or more of these flower oils, which impart what the trade calls 'smoothness' to the mix.

Most precious of all these oils to the perfumer is that obtained from the rose. The species mainly grown for perfumery is the hundred-leaved rose, *Rosa centifolia,* a small, scrubby, rather unimpressive bush. Vast fields of it are grown near Grasse, where the flowers are hand-picked at night when their fragrance is strongest. Because the bushes bloom in May, the attar derived from the French fields is known as *Rose de Mai.* Roses for the perfumer are also grown in Bulgaria, Turkey, and Morocco. Oddly enough, the attar of roses that carried away the prize at the Great Exhibition of 1851 came from Ghazipur, in what was then the Northwest

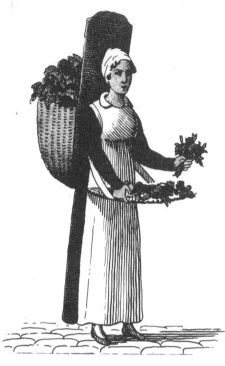

Above: Pinks and roses – a street flower seller cries her wares.

Right: the manager of a perfume factory in Grasse explains the distilling process to a slightly bored Queen Victoria. Along the walls of the factory are paired the stills and condensers, probably at that time made of copper. The still, loaded with petals and water, was boiled up like a huge kettle. The heat broke open the oil-bearing cells in the petals, and steam and petal-oil was carried through the U-shaped tubes into the condenser. In the condenser the steam returned to water, which, being heavier than the oil, settled to the bottom where it could be drained off. The oil left in the condenser was then drawn off into glass flasks.

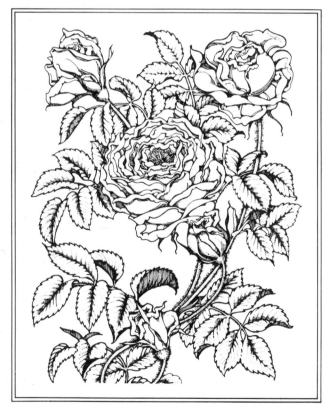

Provinces of India. Although India is not now a major source of high quality attar, there was a time in the 19th century when, according to the *Indian Encyclopaedia*, 'Attar of roses made in Kashmir is considered to be superior to any other; a circumstance not surprising, as . . . the flower is here produced of surpassing fragrance as well as beauty.'

Shakespeare wrote, clumsily for him:

> The rose looks fair, but fairer we it deem
> For that sweet odour which doth in it live.

There are several ways of extracting the 'sweet odour'. Rose water is made by distilling rose petals with water. Rose attar, the absolute, is made by re-distilling rose water and, in a further process, separating off the oil. The scent can also be taken from rose petals by enfleurage.

One of the most famous of rose perfumes is *Red Rose,* made by Floris of London. This was popularized by Edward VII. He was a frequent visitor to the Cavendish Hotel, which was only a few yards from the Floris shop. The Cavendish, a centre of Edwardian social life, had been taken over in 1902 by Rosa Lewis, who was renowned for two things – her quail pudding and her rose perfume, which she bought from Floris. *Red Rose* became Rosa Lewis's trade mark and from her the king caught a liking for it.

Bulgaria produces today some of the best-quality attar of roses used in perfumery. The attar is expensive because the flowers still have to be gathered by hand (*overleaf, left*) and tons of petals are needed to produce the attar by distillation (*overleaf, right*). As a result, synthetic rose oil now frequently replaces natural attar. The rose cultivated commercially in Bulgaria is the Damask rose, *Rosa Damascena*, from which the city of Damascus, ancient capital of Syria, took its name. (The name Syria is also said to be connected with roses; the word is supposed to be derived from *Suri*, meaning 'land of roses'.) The Damask rose has taken over from Bulgaria's native rose, which was the red rose, *Rosa gallica*, one of the oldest plants known to man. It was the red rose that carpeted Cleopatra's and Nero's floors; whose petals were given to Joan of Arc after she had raised the siege of Orleans; and which was the symbol of the House of Lancaster in the Wars of the Roses.

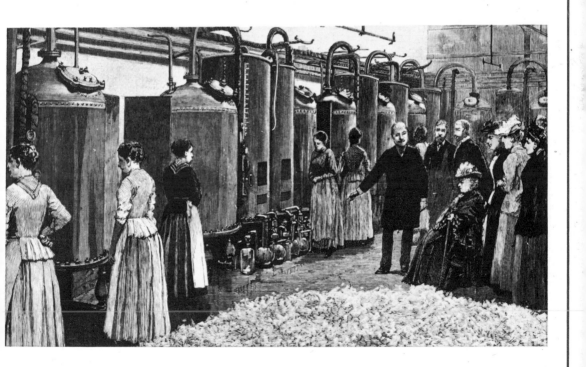

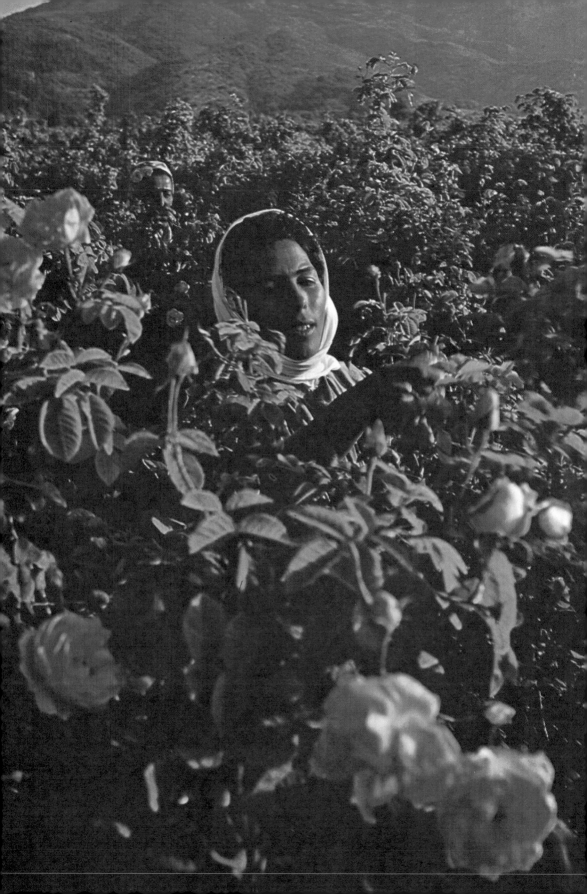

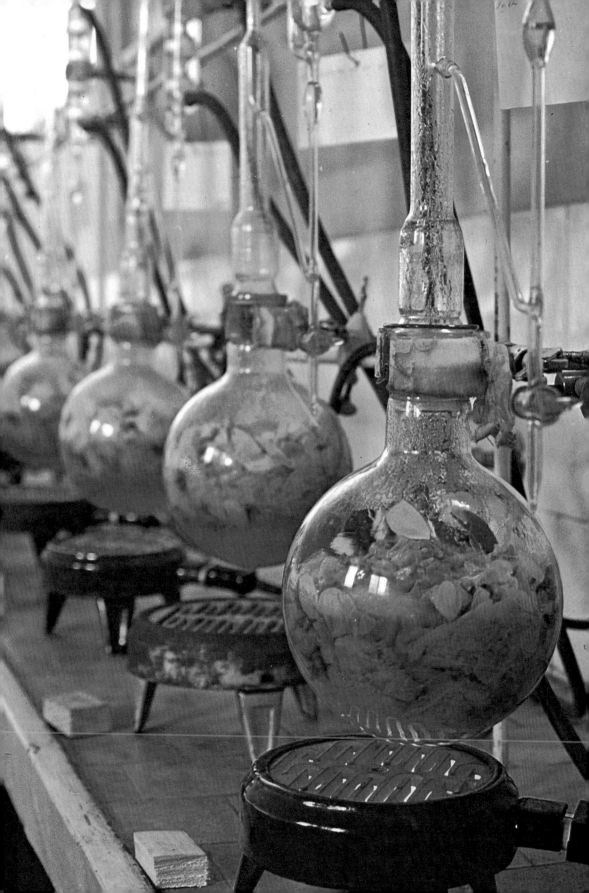

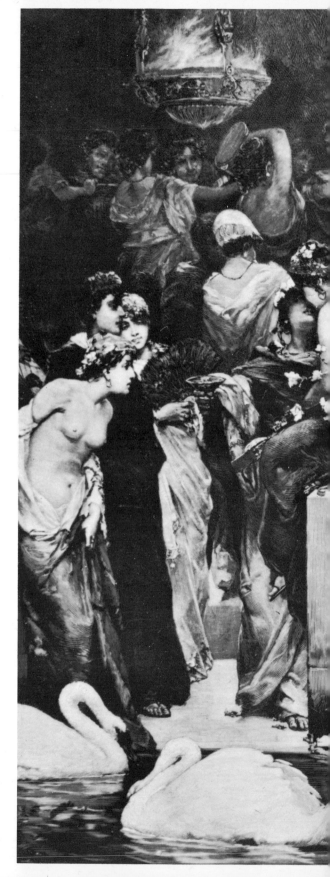

The Roman feasts in honour of Bacchus,
god of wine, became elaborate orgies
that make wife-swapping parties seem
tame and unimaginative in comparison.
Wine, women, and food were essential
ingredients of the bacchanalia, but so,
more surprisingly, were roses. The
Romans were obsessed by the rose.
Rose water perfumed their public baths.
It flowed from fountains in the
emperors' palaces, in the houses of the
rich and powerful, and in the
amphitheatres – where the sweat of the
crowds and the stench from the bloody
arena hung over everything. At banquets
and feasts roses were strewn everywhere;
even the cushions were stuffed with
petals. Women – as in this painting of a
bacchanalian feast by Kobarbinski –
wore roses in their hair. Wine was rose-
scented, and the cure for over-indulgence
in it was rose water. Rose pudding was
a delicacy. Illness was treated with rose
medicine. And, if you were given a love
potion, it would, of course, taste of roses.

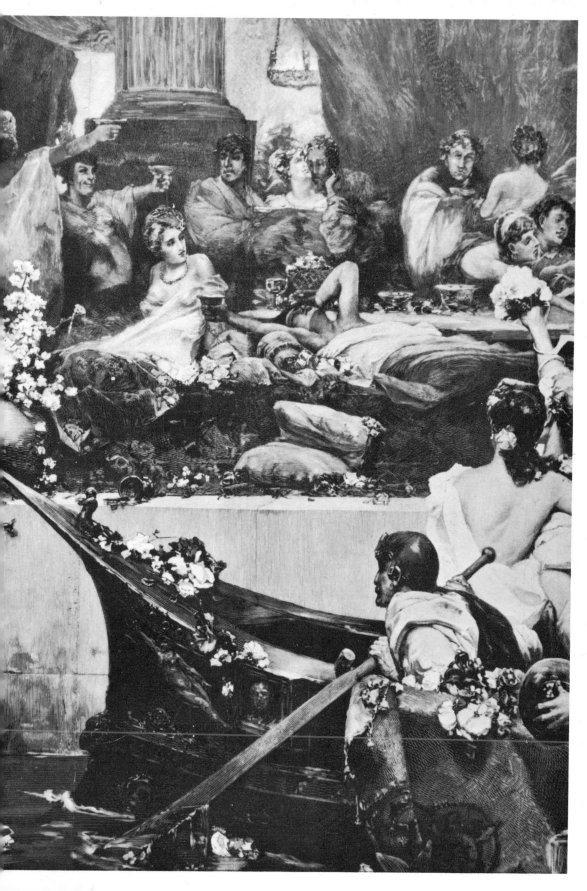

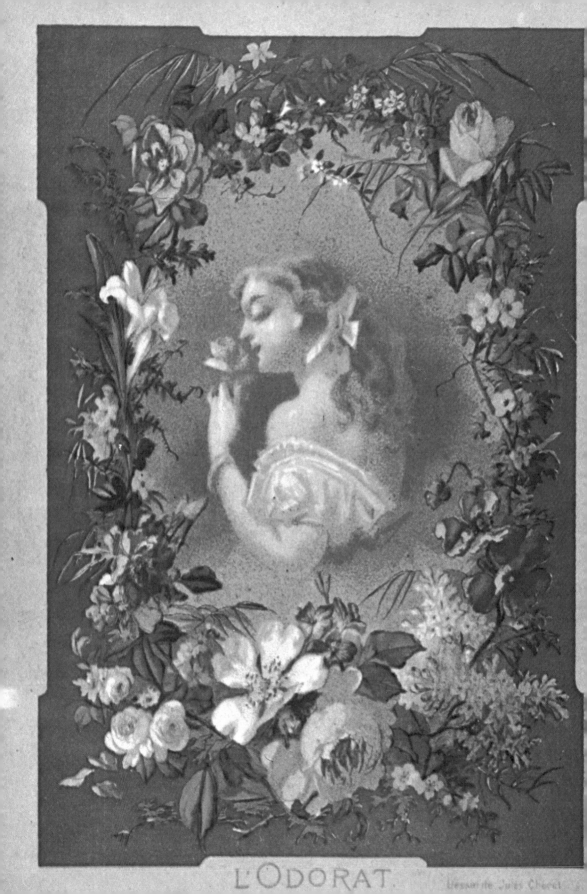

L'ODORAT.

Dessin de Jules Chéret

The first man-made perfumes were a by-product of the discovery of fire. The scents that surrounded early man were natural ones – they were the smells of flowers, trees, animals, and the earth itself. None of these was controllable or usable. The flower that gave off its perfume at dusk could not be switched on at noon; the fresh, scented air after a rainstorm could not be bottled and released at will. Fire was the key that made perfume available. As soon as men noticed that burning woods and gums gave off odours, they had the knowledge to produce perfume when they wanted it. They had only to light a fire.

The memory of these first deliberately created scents is preserved in our word 'perfume', which comes from the Latin *per* meaning 'through', and *fumus* meaning 'smoke'. Every time we use the word to describe the expensively packaged liquids that crowd the shelves of a modern chemist's shop, we are honouring the memory of those unknown men who first appreciated the pleasure of sweet-smelling smoke rising from comforting, crackling fires.

But fire is dangerous as well as comforting. To early man it was a mystical and magical thing, an elemental spirit with a life of its own. Smoke was its sacred child. Moreover, the scented smoke rose into the air and became invisible as though it had become part of the sky itself. It rose into the heavens and never returned. So early man used it as a vehicle or messenger, to carry his prayers to the heavens. Then, because he found it pleasing, he thought that it must also be pleasing to the gods, and he offered it to them in the same way as he offered food and sacrifices – to placate the fickle, powerful beings who controlled his life.

But two things happened – and happened, probably, very early in man's history. The first was the recognition that you don't have to light a fire to make a perfume. Scents could be carried in waters and oils, which could be rubbed on the body. Secondly, man re-appropriated to himself the scented pleasures he offered his gods. Originally, it seems, he anointed his priest-kings. They were on earth; there was no point in sending up to them the smoke of burning incense. Nevertheless, they were divine, and should smell divine. So they were anointed with unguents and oils. Then, as the functions of priests and kings became separated, both were anointed. And the inevitable regression set in. If you anoint the king, why not anoint me, the prince? If you anoint the prince, why not me, his right-hand man? If you anoint the servant of the king, why not me, his courtier? And so on, down the line, until perfume became commonly used in profane as well as sacred circumstances and became the prerogative not only of the gods but of the rich on earth.

By the time recorded history begins, perfume was an accepted and commonplace fact of life. Like clothing, like personal adornments, like cosmetics, it had become part of the social structure. It retained its religious use

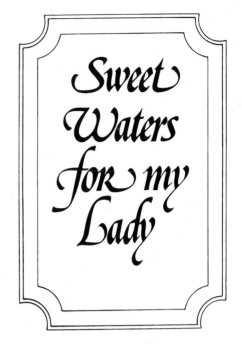

Sweet Waters for my Lady

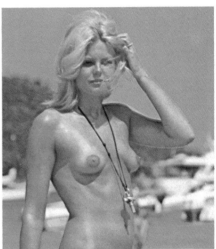

Women's freedom to use perfumes adventurously goes with their social and sexual freedom and runs parallel with experimentation in make-up and with free conventions in dress. The girl shown in the frontispiece to Eugene Rimmel's *Le Livre des Parfums* (*far left*), published in 1864, was limited to light toilet waters and 'innocent' flower scents. The topless girl on the beach at St Tropez (*above*) is free not only to display her body but to perfume it with the strong, natural, 'one-note' scents of the 1970s.

and significance. It still does. Incense is still burned in, for example, Roman Catholic and Greek Orthodox churches. Its royal use remained, and still does. In 1953, Elizabeth II was anointed at her coronation ceremony in Westminster Abbey. But already it was a social status symbol, a trade mark of a leisured, wealthy class. And already it was being used to attract the opposite sex.

When it was that women first began to enhance their sex appeal by perfuming themselves, we simply do not know. It was certainly in prehistoric times. Probably kings stole perfume from the gods, lesser men stole it from kings, and women stole it from men. And we have to remember that the distinction between the sexual use of perfume and the religious use of perfume is one that exists in our minds only. In most religions, in most societies, and at most periods, the sexual act is a form of the act of worship. Perfume went easily enough from temple to bedroom.

In a sense, the history of the personal use of perfume is the history of sophistication. Those societies that were in turn the leaders of civilization were, equally in turn, leaders in their appreciation of the sensuous delights of scent. In the words of Eugene Rimmel, whose *Book of Perfumes*, although more than a century old, is still the standard work on the history of perfume: 'We may say that perfumery was studied and cherished by all the various nations which held in turn the sceptre of civilization. It was transmitted by the Egyptians to the Jews, then to the Assyrians, the Greeks, the Romans, the Arabs, and at last to the modern European nations....'

That this is by and large true is scarcely surprising. Politically powerful nations are wealthy nations, and it is only wealth that permits a life of sufficient leisure and luxury for non-essential refinements like perfume. And sex can become a game, with its rules of courtship and seduction and its toys like perfume and make-up, only when everyday life is essentially secure.

Nonetheless, the historian of scent must beware of falling into the trap of over-simplification that has ensnared Rimmel. The trouble is that the great civilizations he lists are those that are the best-documented. Hence the by-ways of their history, including their use of perfume, are better known to us than those of less-favoured nations. But every society we know of has used scent, and some may have used it more lavishly, more imaginatively, and more glamorously than did, say, the ancient Egyptians or the Greeks.

The historian of perfume has other difficulties. One is that we often know only the scented practices of the great and famous, and although we may with a fair degree of safety generalize from this knowledge – because the great and famous were usually the leaders of fashion – our generalizations may be off target. The more particularly because the public use of scent is often all we have to go on, when it is the intimate details of private lives that would be more to our purpose.

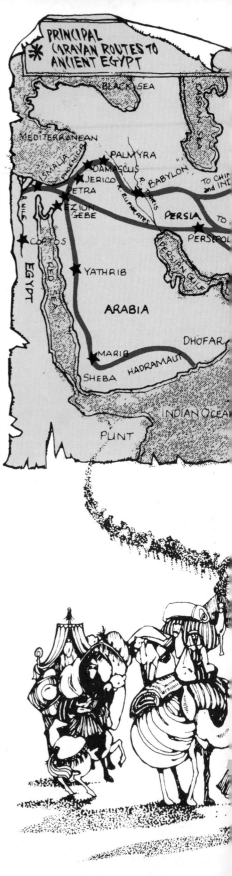

Scent is like make-up. In both cases the usages of the public rooms are different from those of the boudoir, and the usages of the boudoir different from those of the bedroom. Moreover, the usages of the palace are – sometimes – different from those of the brothel.

The civilization that is usually, and probably rightly, credited with being the first to make lavish use of perfume is that of ancient Egypt. We know that the Egyptians used perfume in three ways – in their religious ceremonies, in the embalmment of their dead, and in their private lives. It is hard for us to realize that these three usages were not, in fact, separate. We lead compartmentalized lives. The Egyptians did not. Their religion was an integral part of their everyday life. So was death. To them the journey to the tomb meant not much more than moving house; it was not the traumatic full-stop that we think it today. Nor would they have found it odd that the scent they offered to the gods was also worn by a beautiful woman to make her still more sexually desirable. They had not met the sexual hang-ups that the Christian church later imposed upon Europe. Egyptian gods had a sex life of their own.

In the great temples dedicated to Isis, Osiris, and the other divinities that watched over Egypt, the air was heavy with burning incense. So, too, were the rooms of private houses. And the women of ancient Egypt were as highly scented as a box of spices. Although most of the information that has come down to us is of the ceremonial use of perfume, it is probably true that the private consumption of scent in Egypt was greater than the religious. The Egyptians were a hygienically minded people who believed that cleanliness was next to godliness. It was they who invented the elaborate system of baths that the Romans took over and became famous for. And Egyptian women made more frequent and more sybaritic use of the bath than Roman women ever did. Egyptian men made as much of a fetish of women's soft, pale, scented skin as modern Western man does of shapely breasts and legs. So after her bath the rich Egyptian woman would lie naked while her slave girls massaged fragrant oils and ointments into her skin

Overleaf: the setting is King Solomon's magnificent palace in Jerusalem; the time is somewhen in the 10th century B.C.; the occasion is the arrival of the queen of Sheba. Nowadays, most summit meetings are about oil; this one – the most famous and glamorous of them all – was about perfume. The kingdom of Sheba, in the south of Arabia, grew frankincense and myrrh and its whole economy depended upon the sale of these two products. Egypt was the main market. Year in and year out, the camel trains of Sheba plodded along the Incense Road (see map), carrying their precious cargoes to the land of the pharaohs. This was a high-risk trade. Whole camel trains might be hijacked by marauding tribesmen. Less dramatically, they were wide open to pilferage. Spices and incense were the sneak-thief's dream: they had small bulk and high unit value. One way and another, losses – in men and goods – could be high on the long, slow, parched journey. But the rewards for a successful merchant could be correspondingly great, and without this hard-earned income Sheba would be bankrupt. Now the Incense Road was threatened by the expanded empire of King Solomon. The Sheban caravans had to run the gauntlet of the Israelite army, whose chariots straddled the northern section of the Road. It was so important to keep the Road open that the queen of Sheba decided that she must be her own ambassador to Solomon. She set off by camel train on the arduous 2,000-mile journey to Jerusalem, where Solomon lived with 'seven hundred wives and three hundred concubines'. The queen was glamorous enough to be more than a match for even this amount of competition. She overwhelmed the bemused Solomon, flattering him outrageously and presenting him with myrrh, frankincense, gold, jewels, and herself. Solomon succumbed. The queen returned to Sheba smugly triumphant. Not only had she secured the freedom of the Incense Road; she had earned a bonus – the contract to supply Solomon's empire with incense.

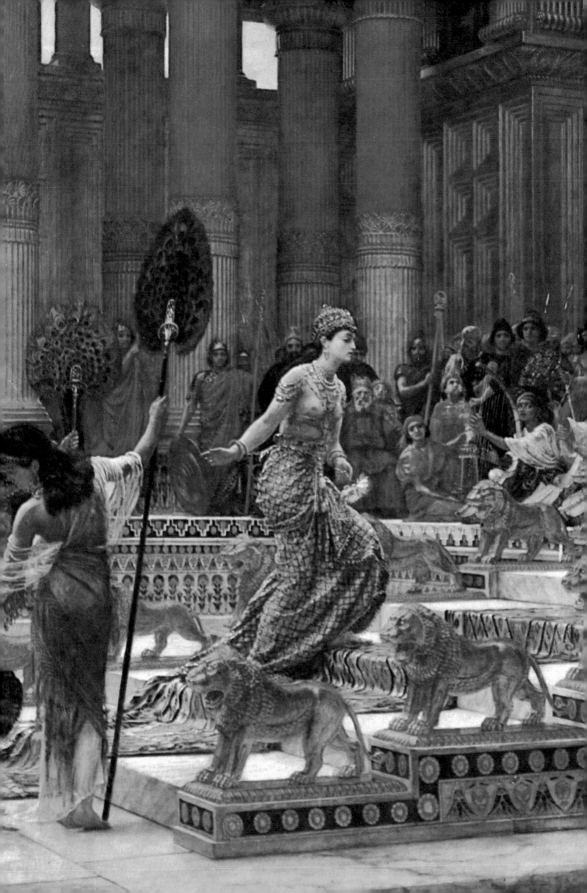

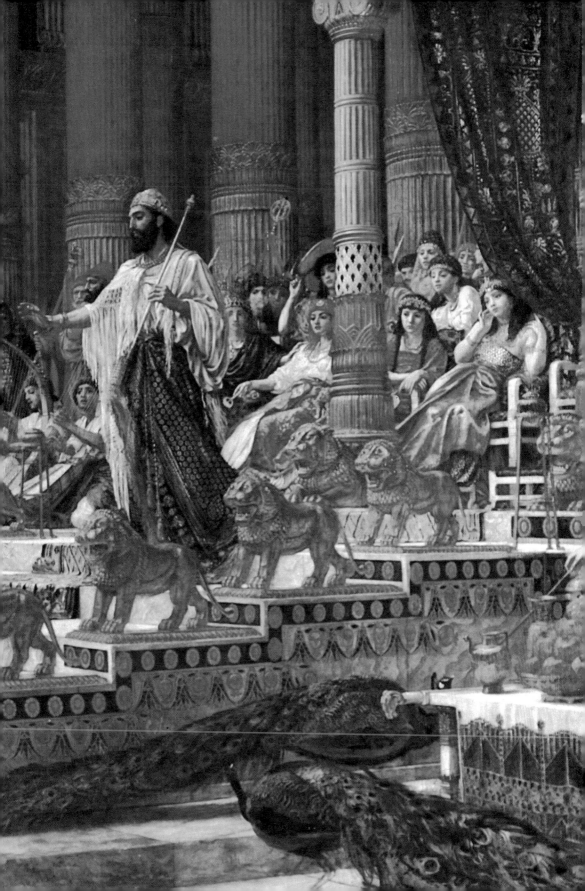

The unguents used for this were at first prepared and sold by the priests, who found manufacturing perfumery a lucrative side-line and who were thus, as far as we know, the earliest retail perfumers. Some of the ingredients they used to make these scented toilet preparations were home produced, like origanum and bitter almonds, but most had to be imported. Myrrh and frankincense, for example, came from Arabia. The cost of these imports was enormous – a burden supportable only by an immensely wealthy nation.

Upper-class women of ancient Egypt, lucky enough to be the rich citizens of a rich nation, enjoyed a total social freedom. Their life was a luxurious social round. They were beautifully dressed, beautifully coiffured, beautifully made up, and lavishly perfumed. We cannot use the word 'beautiful' of their perfumes, because Egyptian perfumes were too hot and spicy for our tastes. Cinnamon and nutmeg were both popular perfume ingredients. So were almonds, frankincense, myrrh, sweet rushes, laurel, and juniper. Probably, too, the animal smells of musk and civet were used in Egyptian perfumes – both obtained from Ethiopia.

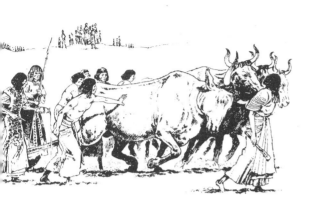

The ancient Egyptians believed that the dead still needed their earthly bodies in the after-life. They went to great lengths to preserve the bodies of their dead, evolving over the centuries elaborate techniques of mummification. The mummification industry swallowed up vast quantities of scent products and a huge labour force. The morticians and embalmers supported an army of parts suppliers – the craftsmen who made the surgical instruments, the containers, the bandages, and the ointments for the funeral parlours of Egypt. Only the rich were mummified – the body of the ordinary labourer was simply dumped unceremoniously in a communal pit. At the other end of the scale, the pharaoh or high official received the full treatment in the embalming shop. His brain was pulled out through his nose. His heart, liver, lungs, and intestines were cut out, the resulting cavities filled with cassia and myrrh, and the body stitched together again. The removed organs were placed in jars containing scented preservatives. The body was drained of any remaining blood and left to dehydrate in a bath of natron. After about seventy days it was removed, rubbed dry, and given cosmetic attention – linen pads were inserted under the skin to plump out the cheeks and remould the shrunken limbs. Finally the corpse was wrapped in hundreds of yards of linen bandages impregnated with scented ointments (*left*).

There were quicker and cheaper processes available – in one, the body was simply dried out in natron and pickled in salt. There were degrees of splendour in the funeral procession too. The rich man's mummy was placed in a fragrant cedarwood coffin and borne on an ornate funeral sledge (*above*) to the tomb that was to be its dwelling house. There the dead man was surrounded by all the everyday objects of his earthly life – some tombs, fitted with all mod. cons., even provided a mummy lavatory. In the early days of Egypt, slaves and servants were also provided for the dead man. They were those of his attendants who, at his death, had 'volunteered' to poison themselves so that they could be buried beside him.

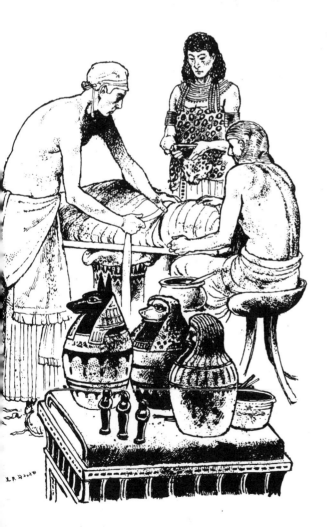

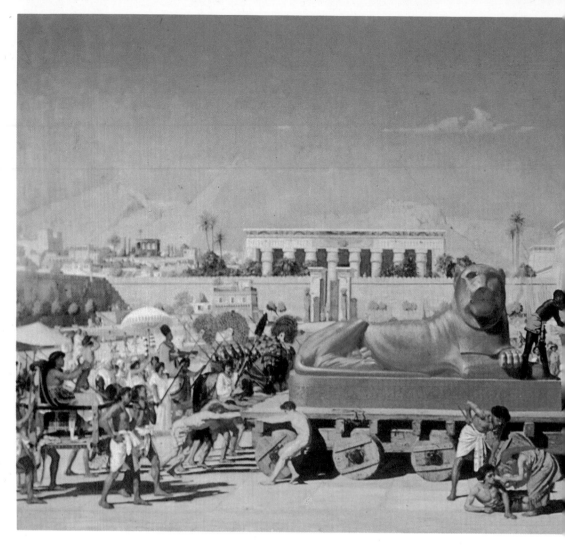

In Sir Edward Poynter's painting *Israel in Egypt* (1867), a Jewish labour gang, under the whips of Egyptian overseers, hauls a huge statue to its site. During their long captivity in Egypt the Jews learned from their conquerors the arts of perfumery. They formed part of the work force the Egyptians needed for their great building projects and, as they went about their drudgery, they saw at first hand how the Egyptians used incense and ointments in their temples, tombs, and homes. The Egyptians were, at all times, great builders. Their temple at Karnak is still the largest religious building the world has ever known. Just one of its chambers, the Hypostyle Hall, covers 54,000 square feet — roughly the area of Canterbury Cathedral. But the Egyptians devoted perhaps their greatest energies to the building of their pyramids and tombs. Many pharaohs spent the greater part of their lives in

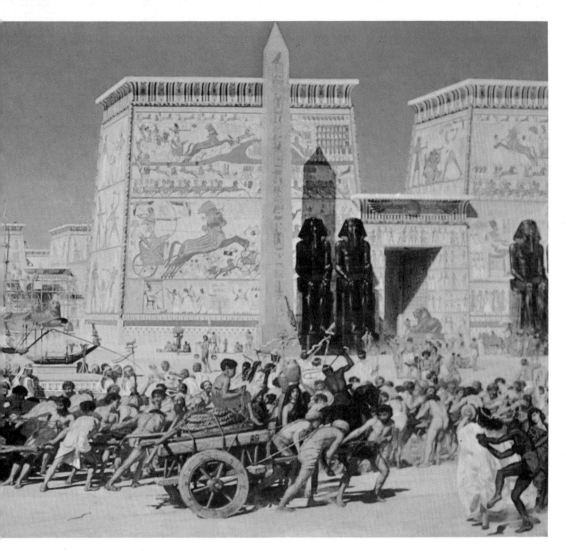

planning the construction and overseeing the erection of the tombs that would house their bodies after death. Much of this time was spent in trying to invent ways to foil the tomb robbers. Great riches were buried with a pharaoh — an eternal temptation to the thief. Among the crowds who watched the funeral procession of a pharaoh there were always men licking their lips at the sight of the treasures that accompanied him to the grave. The perfumes and the jewels were particularly tempting — they were profitable, high-value goods that could easily be disposed of to a fence. Devious and complicated security systems were incorporated in Egyptian tombs to try and defeat the robbers. The pyramids should have given protection by sheer bulk. The body of the pharaoh Cheops was surrounded in its Great Pyramid by five million tons of stone — enough, Napoleon calculated, to build a ten-foot-high

wall round France. But over eighty pyramids were built, and every one was looted by robbers. Underground tombs were no answer either. They incorporated mazes of passage-ways, dead ends, and concealed entrances that were meant to be found — they simply led to complicated systems of empty rooms. Their corridors were blocked by portcullises, strong sealed doors, and huge stone plugs. But the robbers always won. The pharaohs never beat them, mainly because the Egyptian authorities never got to the root of the robbery problem. This was, simply, that most tomb robberies were the outcome of a collaboration between an outside gang of thieves and an inside informer. In almost every case, the inside man was the priest who had been charged with the upkeep and security of the tomb. No one knew better than he the way to the treasures he guarded.

The consumption of perfumes in ancient Egypt was certainly immense, but it is impossible to quantify. We have some clues. We know, for example, something of the glamorous ostentation with which one queen of Egypt, Cleopatra, used perfume. Cleopatra's meeting with Antony on her scent-sodden barge is still part of our folklore over 2,000 years later. But this is a scrap of history preserved by strokes of luck. A hundred years after Antony's death a Greek wrote his biography; that biography survived to be translated 1,500 years later into French; from the French an Englishman made an English translation; and from that translation Shakespeare created lines, some of which we have already quoted, that made the occasion unforgettable:

> For her own person
> It beggar'd all description: she did lie
> In her pavillion, – cloth-of-gold of tissue, –
> O'er-picturing that Venus where we see
> The fancy out-work nature ... From the barge
> A strange invisible perfume hits the sense
> Of the adjacent wharfs.

But by the time of Cleopatra the great days of Egypt were long past and Cleopatra, herself more Greek than Egyptian, ruled a dying empire. It has been said that in her time the Egyptian taste for perfume reached its peak, but this is unlikely to be true. Shakespeare has impressed us too much and Cleopatra has become one of the sex-goddesses of history. She has overshadowed unjustly the women of the courts of the earlier pharaohs. Queen Nefertiti, for example, wife of the pharaoh Amenhotep IV, who lived over a thousand years before Cleopatra, has no legend to immortalize her and no Shakespeare to make her come alive to us. But this most beautiful and mysterious of all queens – whose name means, literally, 'the lovely stranger' – would certainly have been more lavishly, and perhaps more subtly, perfumed than Cleopatra.

The Egyptians taught the whole ancient world how to use scent. In particular, and by direct contact, they taught the Jews. The Jewish people had used perfume, at least in their religious rites, since the very earliest times, but it seems to have been the captivity in Egypt that initiated them into the more sophisticated personal use of scents. Moses decreed severe penalties against anyone using holy oils and incense for private purposes. The fact that the prohibition was necessary proves that perfume was being taken from the temples to become a personal indulgence. It perhaps suggests that it was a new habit of the Jewish people. It is unlikely that the ban on perfumes was effective. Throughout history governments have tried to control cosmetics, personal adornment, hair styles, and artificial aids to beauty. None of these attempts has succeeded for long. Jewish women, like all other women, used perfume as a cosmetic just as their tutors, the Egyptians, did. The virgins offered to King Xerxes so that he could select from them

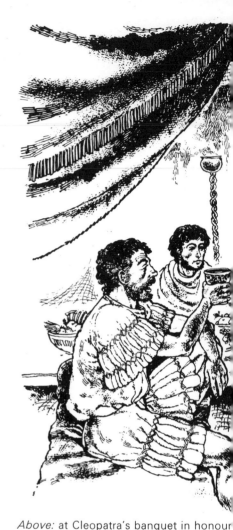

Above: at Cleopatra's banquet in honour of Mark Antony the whole floor was covered to the depth of several feet with scented roses. There was a purpose behind this and other extravagances in Cleopatra's entertainment of Antony. Cleopatra had had hopes of sitting with Caesar on the throne of a united Romano-Egyptian empire. She had been living with Caesar in Rome, had had a son by him, and seemed set to found with him a new and powerful dynasty. But Caesar had been murdered and Cleopatra's hopes had died with him. Now she saw Mark Antony as Caesar's successor, the new master of the Roman world. She determined to carry on with

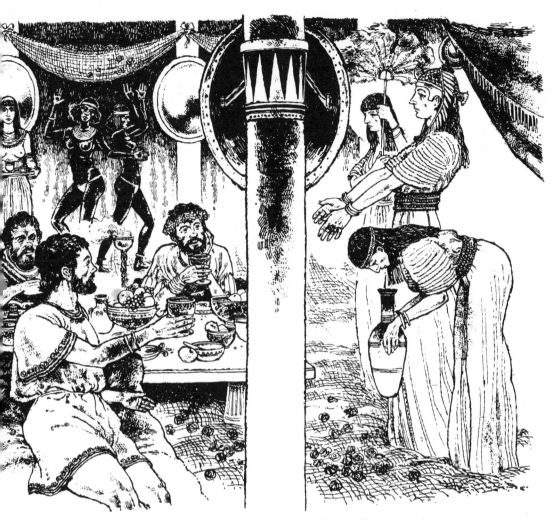

her plans, simply substituting Antony for Caesar. Her ambition was political as well as personal. Egypt was nominally an independent kingdom, although it was protected by Roman legions. If Cleopatra failed to secure an alliance with Antony, her country was likely to be mopped up and to become just another Roman province. She set out to captivate Antony. She had to impress him personally, to show herself as a suitable consort. Equally important, she had to impress upon him the power and wealth of Egypt – to demonstrate that Egypt was worthy of partnership with Rome. Much as a business man today tries to impress another by giving him

an expensive lunch, Cleopatra wined and dined Antony. She was a mistress of the arts of hospitality and she ruled over a court that knew refinements of luxury beyond the experience of Rome. She gave this banquet in the saloon of her state barge, which was more a floating palace than a boat. The carpet of roses was held in position by nets fixed to the side walls. The air was heavy with incense. As a final touch, Cleopatra dissolved a huge pearl in vinegar and drank it down – thus neatly making the point that a pearl that would have been priceless in Rome was in her rich country nothing more than a cheap, expendable bauble.

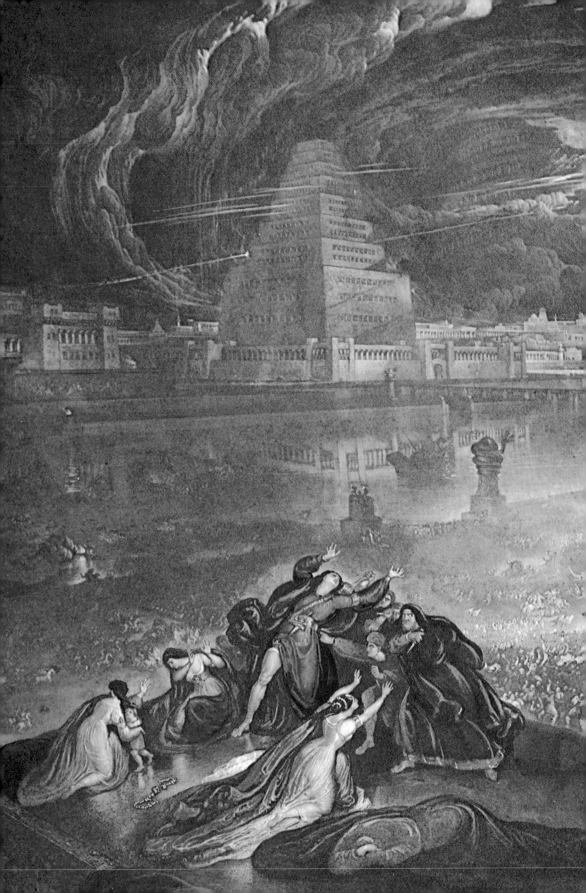

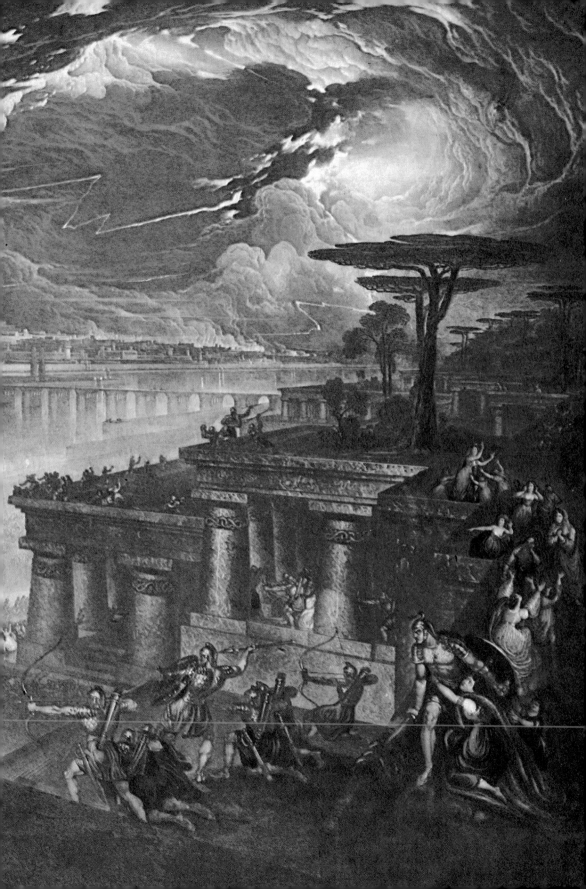

Previous page: The Destruction of Babylon, by the 19th-century British artist John Martin. The city of Babylon was sacked and razed to the ground by Sennacherib in 689 B.C. But it is the Wrath of God, not Sennacherib, who is the destroyer in Martin's painting. The picture is mythological, not historical. Babylon entered into Christian mythology because of its reputation for luxury and dissolute living. Like Sodom and Gomorrah, it became a synonym for sin. Martin has chosen to depict the city as it looked after it had been rebuilt under Nebuchadnezzar. In the right foreground are the famous Hanging Gardens of Babylon, which were not 'hanging' at all. They were roof gardens laid out on balconies. Across the water is the great ziggurat, or Tower of Babel, the greatest wonder of all in a city that Herodotus said 'surpasses in splendour any city of the known world'. The ziggurat was as old as Babylon itself. Sennacherib managed only to damage it and Nebuchadnezzar had it repaired. It was a colossal stepped platform – in reality about 300 feet wide at its base and some 200 feet high – built in seven stages. On the top was a temple to the sun god, Baal. The ziggurat was a solid structure built of sun-dried bricks. To stop the bricks crumbling under the sheer weight of the tower, layers of reed-matting were added to act like steel-rod reinforcements in a modern concrete building. An outside flight of steps led to the second storey; from there on worshippers had to ascend by ramps. Inside the temple at the summit was a gold statue of Baal and an enormous altar, also of gold, on which frankincense was burned – one idea of the ziggurat being that it reached high into the heavens so that smoke from the incense would more quickly reach the god.

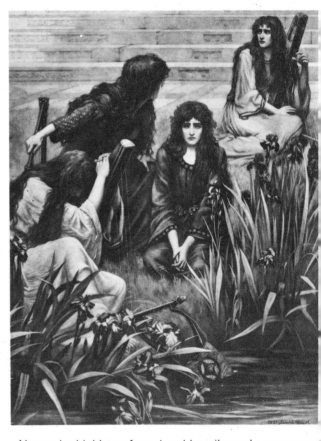

Above: the highly perfumed and heavily made-up women of Babylon were reputed to be the most beautiful and desirable of the ancient world. An Egyptian pharaoh, Amenhotep III, perhaps wanting to find out the truth of this for himself, once demanded a Babylonian woman for his harem. His request went unanswered – he was too mean to send an Egyptian woman to the king of Babylon in exchange. Babylonian women lived in a free-spending, pleasure-loving city and they had the pick of exotic perfumes at their disposal. Babylon – situated where a main perfume route from the East crossed the Euphrates – was a great international scent market.

a replacement for his disobedient queen, Vashti, underwent a year of purification and beautification before being presented to the king: 'to wit, six months with oil of myrrh, and six months with sweet odours'. The winner of that particular beauty competition was Esther.

Another Jewish heroine was Judith, who saved her native city by seducing Holofernes, the Assyrian commander of the force that besieged it, and killing him as he lay on his bed in drunken exhaustion. She, too, used perfume to aid her. 'And she washed her body and anointed herself with the best ointment . . . and adorned herself with all her ornaments. And the Lord also gave her more beauty . . . so that she appeared to all men's eyes incomparably lovely.'

The story of Judith is probably historical romance, but Holofernes certainly existed. He was one of Nebuchadnezzar's generals. Certainly, too, he would have expected his women to be perfumed. The Assyrians were a perfume-oriented people. The magnificent pleasure cities of Nineveh and Babylon were redolent with scent. Babylonian scents were world-famous and the city was the chief market for eastern perfumes. Its Hanging Gardens, created by Nebuchadnezzar to amuse his homesick wife Amytes, were designed to please the sense of smell as much as the sense of sight. The gardens were thickly planted with smeet-smelling shrubs and flowers. Amytes' favourite spot was said to have been a bower of scented roses and lilies.

Assyrian women, famous throughout the Middle East for their beauty and sex appeal, perfumed themselves, according to Herodotus, with the most expensive scents. Like the Egyptians, they could afford costly imports. There still exists a clay tablet from Babylon, dating from about 1800 B.C., that is an order form for 'imported oil of cedar, myrrh, and cypress'. Mostly, this would have been used to oil the women's bodies and their hair – Assyrian women evolved some of the most elaborate hair styles that the world has known. But Herodotus also tells us that they 'bruised with a stone the wood of the cypress, cedar, and frankincense and poured water upon it until it became of the desired consistency. With this they anointed the body and the face. . . .' The liquid seems to have been applied like a face pack, but to the whole body. It was left on for some time and then removed, leaving the skin soft, scented, and, hopefully, free from blemish.

This sort of body pack was rare in the ancient world. Most perfumes were oils or wines, scented with flowers or gums, that were simply rubbed in all over the body. The Greeks went one step further, and used a different perfume for each part of the body. A lover might find his mistress's breasts smelling differently from her neck and her thighs differently from her knees. But perhaps this was just a passing fad, for the difficulty of finding non-clashing scents must have been enormous. Greek women could never have been ready in time.

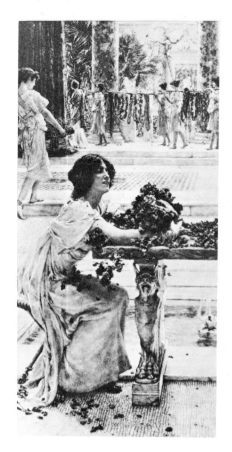

Above: a 19th-century romantic painter's view of ancient Greece – Sir Lawrence Alma-Tadema's *Flowers*. The Greeks were always fond of flower garlands like those carried by the girls in the background.

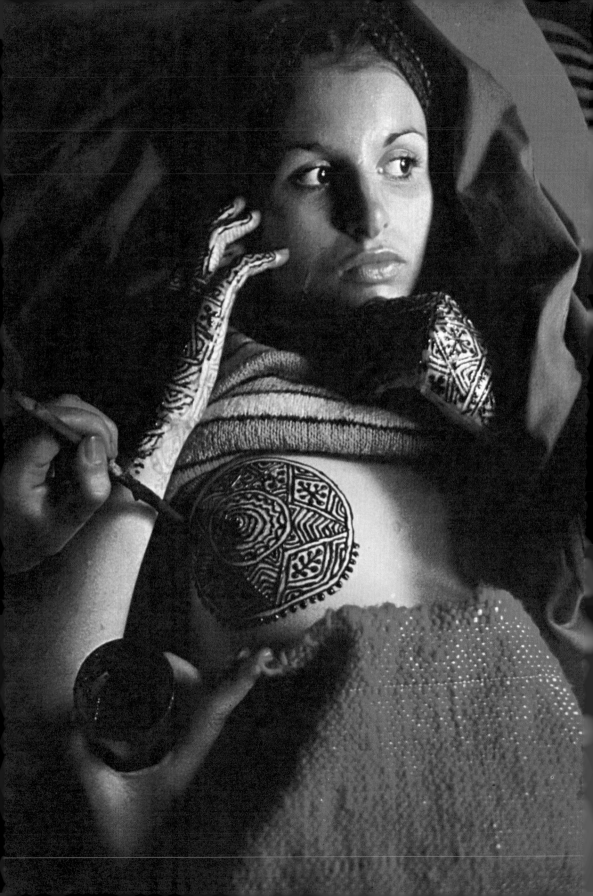

They had a great number of perfumes to choose from. Apollonius of Herophila, who wrote an early treatise on perfumery, listed some of the 'best buys' of ancient Greece: 'The iris is best at Elis and at Cyzicus; the perfume made from roses is most excellent at Pharselis, and that made at Naples and Capua is also very fine. That made from crocus is most perfect from Soli in Cilicia and at Rhodes. The essence of spikenard is best at Tarsus, and of vine leaves at Cyprus and Adramyttium. The best perfume from marjoram and from apples comes from Cos.'

On the whole the Greeks kept their women firmly in their place, which was the kitchen and the nursery. At very few periods did Greek women have the same freedom as had the women of Egypt. Perhaps as a result, respectable women of Greece were neither great nor imaginative users of cosmetics. They left that to the *hetairi*, the courtesans of Greece, who went in for very elaborate make-up, including an eye-paint that has a very 1970s look. The *hetairi*, whose bodies were their livelihood, also made a very liberal use of scent. We have a description of the toilet of one successful courtesan, whose slave girls first massaged her from head to toe, then placed her in a scented bath, dried her with swan's feathers, and finally rubbed her whole body with 'scented oils from the East'. Other *hetairi* perfumed their breath by holding scented liquid in their mouths and rolling it around with their tongues – a trick that was used again by London prostitutes in the mid-18th century.

This would have been behaviour too extreme and overtly sexual for the respectable Greek woman, but she would nonetheless not have objected to perfumes as such. She would have thought them perfectly acceptable. Indeed, more than acceptable. The Greeks looked upon perfume as of divine origin and as an attribute of the gods. The early Greek poets surrounded all their goddesses with fragrance. Homer, for example, describes Juno's preparations to meet Venus:

Here first she bathes, and round her body pours
Soft oils of fragrance and ambrosial showers,
The winds, perfumed, the balmy gale conveys
Through heaven, through earth, and all the aerial ways.

Venus herself was, of course, exquisitely perfumed and it was through her that perfumes reached mortal women. The secrets of Venus's fragrance were revealed by the nymph Oenone to Paris, and he passed them on to the legendary beautiful Helen of Troy. She taught them to her countrywomen on her return from Troy.

But perfume in Greece very quickly passed from the world of the gods to the world of commerce. Hundreds of perfumers set up shop in Athens. Some gave their own names to particular scents, and jealously guarded their trade marks. Megallium, for example, was the product of a high-class perfumer called Megallus:

And say you are bringing her such unguents
As old Megallus never did compound.

he henna plant provides us with the perfume cyprinum and also gives us one of the oldest known cosmetics. Today most of us think of henna only as a hair dye. It is still used in modern hair salons for tinting and as a medium to carry other hair preparations. This is because it is safe – it coats the hair but does not penetrate it. But henna has other cosmetic uses. It is an effective anti-perspirant. Perhaps this is why for many centuries Egyptian and Indian women have dyed with henna the soles of their feet and the palms of their hands – both areas of heavy perspiration. (We are told of an Indian princess of the classical period who employed a maidservant whose sole duty was to follow her to the bath and wipe the red footprints from the wet floor.) Moslem women also use henna to paint intricate designs (*left*) on certain parts of their bodies for certain special occasions. A bride is decorated for her first – and only her first – wedding. And many Moslem women decorate themselves for the festival of the Moslem New Year.

Another perfumer was a household word to the Athens jet-set:

> I left the man in Peron's shop just now
> Dealing for ointment; when he has agreed,
> He'll bring you cinnamon and spikenard essence.

Shops like Peron's sold a variety of perfumes. Writing in the early years of the third century B.C., Theophrastus, a disciple of Aristotle, gives some idea of the range of scents available:

'Perfumes are compounded from various parts of plants – flowers, leaves, roots, wood, fruit, and gum – and in most cases the perfume is made from a mixture of several parts. Rose and gillyflower perfumes are made from the flowers . . . made from leaves are those culled from myrtle and dropwort. . . . From roots are made the scents named from iris, spikenard, and sweet marjoram.' Theophrastus also mentions an 'Egyptian perfume', which was probably kyphi or a Greek imitation of it.

The Romans, particularly in Imperial times, copied the Greek love of scent – even adopting the Greek fashion of using a different perfume on different parts of the body. In the time of Ovid, who was roughly contemporary with Christ, Rome had almost as many perfumers' shops as Athens at its peak. In Capua, a pleasure-city like Pompeii, the perfumers occupied a whole street. Many of the flower essences that made up the bulk of their stock were home-produced, but most were imported from Egypt and Arabia.

Roman women had on their toilet tables three types of perfumes: solid unguents, liquid unguents with an oil base, and powders. We know the names of some of the liquid perfumes. There was *rhodium,* made from roses; *melinum,* made from quince flowers; and *narcissinum,* made from narcissus blossoms. More complicated – and more expensive – unguents were *nardinum,* whose ingredients included spikenard and myrrh, and *susinum,* which included lilies, honey, saffron, and myrrh.

All these fragrances – and many more – were available to the Roman woman after her bath. In the early days the Romans anointed their bodies after bathing only with pure olive oil. Later, however, men and women alike used oils mixed with various, mainly floral, perfumes. The use of scented oils, ointments, and pomades became so popular in the Roman empire that their manufacture was a flourishing industry. It was an industry that produced cheap perfumes for the relatively poor, as well as expensive ones for the rich. The composition of these cheap scents is unknown to us, but we know of their existence from a throwaway line by the first-century poet Martial, who complained of a mean host who drenched himself in an expensive scent called *Cosmos,* but offered his guests a cheap perfume that 'a starving prostitute would disdain to use'.

Poppaea, the sexy and dissolute wife of the emperor Nero, who, according to Tacitus, 'had every asset except goodness', was in her time the leader of upper-

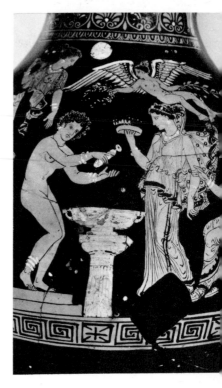

Above: a Roman red-figure vase of the 4th century B.C. showing a bride being prepared for the marriage ceremony. Her limbs will be anointed with aromatic oils. Already her slave attendant is pouring the oil from the perfume bottle.

class fashion in cosmetics and perfumes. She invented a scented face cream, which was known as Poppaea's cream'. She kept her skin soft and white by bathing daily in asses' milk to which scent had been added – a herd of 500 she-asses was maintained especially to fill her bath. Not many Roman women could have competed with that, but Poppaea's cream must have been as much the status symbol of the rich woman as was *Chanel No. 5* almost two thousand years later.

The cream retained its popularity – because of its imperial associations – longer than most perfumes. Fashions changed in the ancient world as they do today – and almost as quickly. Although the mass media did not exist to sweep fashion changes through every layer of society almost overnight, the communities in which people lived were smaller and more intimate and news travelled fast within them. No doubt there were times in Rome when no top people would use *melinum* and everybody who was anybody used *nardinum*. Certainly there was a time when it wasn't done to smell of anything but roses. That the fashion didn't last we know from Petronius, who wrote in the time of Poppaea:

> *Wives are out of fashion. Mistresses are in.*
> *Rose leaves are dated,*
> *Now cinnamon's the thing.*

And no doubt Roman society took the hint. Petronius had spoken, and cinnamon became the thing even if it wasn't before.

With the fall of the Roman empire, power and perfume passed to the Eastern empire. The splendour of Byzantium was a scented splendour. Its palaces were redolent with all the fragrances of the east and its ports the centres of the scent trade. Then the crescent replaced the cross over Constantinople, and the Arabs in their turn became the perfumers of the world. And it was left to them to make the most important discovery in the history of perfumes. It was alcohol.

The discovery that the aroma of plants could be extracted and preserved by a process of distillation made possible the perfumes that we know today. Before then scents had to be incorporated either into a wine base or into an oily mess. Most of the women of the ancient world would have smelled horrible to us – too spicy, too sickly, and probably too rancid. However gorgeous they may have looked, Helen of Troy, Cleopatra, and Poppaea would have smelled so appallingly to a Western man of today that they would have reduced him to total impotence.

The Arabs had long known, as had other peoples, scented resins, oils, and spices. They had long traded in frankincense and myrrh and other fragrant gums. But they had no way of satisfactorily preserving in a long-lasting medium the true scents of flowers. They were not, of course, alone in this. The rose perfumes of Greece and Rome must have smelled of anything but roses. The man who made the breakthrough was the

Below: the Trojan horse – the trick that, according to legend, enabled the Greeks to end ten years of siege, capture the city of Troy, and return to her people the beautiful Helen, wife of the king of Sparta. The Greeks ascribed a divine origin to perfumes and believed that the art of perfumery was taught to mortals by the gods. Their myth had it that Paris, son of the king of Troy, married Oenone, nymph-daughter of the river god Celsen, and was taught by her the secrets of perfumery. When, later, Paris carried off Helen of Troy, he passed on the secrets to her and she brought them to Greece when she returned from Troy.

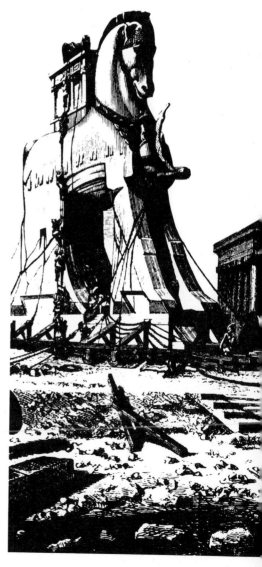

great physician, philosopher, and scientist Avicenna, who lived from 980 to 1036. By inventing distilling he invented the modern perfume. He chose for his first experiments the Arab's favourite flower, the rose, and he succeeded in extracting from it a perfume that is still a favourite all over the world – rose water.

Rose water came to Europe at the time of the Crusades. Christian knights became fascinated with things eastern and, particularly, with eastern women. The idea of the harem, of women whose whole existence was devoted to being indolently attractive to their master, captured their imaginations – and has haunted the erotic dreams of Western men ever since. Hopefully, returning knights brought home to their ladies the perfumes of the harem. Or, more commonly, perfumes that they had been persuaded were of the harem. There were plausible salesmen even then. *Eau de chypre,* brought back by many a gullible Crusader, had no connection with Cyprus, nothing in common with the great classical perfumes from the island, and had never seen the inside of a harem. But it became a symbol of forbidden sexuality and was immensely fashionable in Europe round about the middle of the 12th century. It seems to have been some sort of flower water.

This was the beginning of a reintroduction of perfumes into Europe on a scale that had not been known since Roman times. The Crusaders were only one element in this resurgence; rapidly increasing wealth was a more important factor. Most of these perfumes were at first imported from the Middle East, but local business talent quickly got into the act. By the time the 12th century ended manufacturing perfumers were supplying their own products to the women of France; they were important and numerous enough to be granted a charter by the king, Philip Augustus, in 1190. For some time these perfumers, and others in Europe, were mainly copyists. They merely reproduced the traditional scents of the Middle East and probably had the same sort of reputation as imitators as did Japanese industry immediately after World War II.

The first post-Roman European invention of a perfume seems to have been that of lavender water, traditionally credited to St Hildegarde, a Benedictine abbess more noted for her miraculous visions than for any interest in the cosmetic arts. If the invention was hers it must have been made some time in the 12th century; she died in 1179. Lavender water was made in England very early on and Mitcham, in Surrey, became famous for its lavender. The water was made also in Germany and in France, where, in about 1370, Charles V had lavender planted in the gardens of the Louvre so that he could ensure a supply of the water. His son, Charles VI, was also fond of lavender and had baskets of it hung in his palaces to sweeten the air.

Lavender water has retained its popularity right up to our own day. Another European toilet water had a

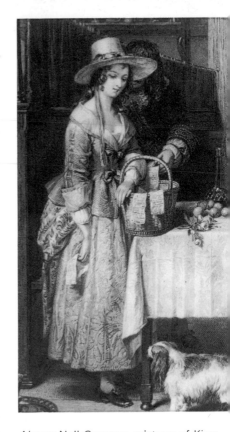

Above: Nell Gwynne, mistress of King Charles II – who remained, if not faithful, at least loyal to her until his death. When Charles was recalled to the throne in 1660, he brought back to the English court and the English leisured classes a frivolity and luxury that had been suppressed in Cromwellian times. Perfumes and cosmetics became the playthings of the Restoration court beauties. At one time an orange scent became popular – perhaps as a sly comment on Nell Gwynne's poor and rather disreputable beginnings.

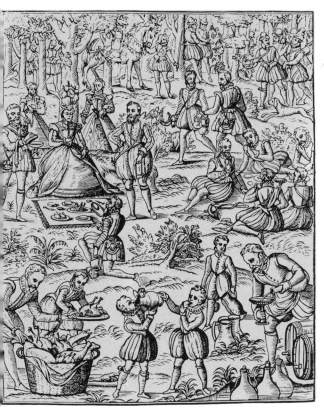

Left: a contemporary woodcut of Elizabeth I enjoying an elaborate picnic with her courtiers. Elizabeth had a passion for scents (it was said of her that 'the sharpness of her nose was equalled only by the sharpness of her tongue') and the courtiers who surrounded her were also highly perfumed. This was partly to please the queen, but the Elizabethans' thickly padded clothes, which were rarely laundered, made it particularly necessary for them to hide their unwashed smell with artificial scents.

Madame de Pompadour (*below*), mistress of Louis XV of France, was one of the leaders in the search for a new and fresher flower fashion in scents. Her favourite flower was the hyacinth, which she ordered to be used indoors during winter and spring, when few other scented flowers were in bloom. She succeeded not only in filling her rooms with fragrance but in making hyacinths so popular that their price rocketed to unprecedented heights.

life almost equally long. 'Hungary water' first began to appear as part of the cosmetic armoury of European ladies in about 1370. Distilled from rosemary, it was the eau de Cologne of the late Middle Ages and it was still in use in Victorian times. It is said to have been prepared first by Queen Elizabeth of Hungary. The story goes that an old hermit told the queen the secret of its preparation, and that she became so desirable through its use that men were still besotted with her when she was seventy. When she was seventy-two, she was so beautiful that the king of Poland found her irresistible and asked for her hand in marriage.

In England the great period for perfumes was that of Elizabeth I. The fashion for the lavish application of scent was brought to England from Italy, which in the 16th century led the Western world in perfumery. France, which later became the world's perfume centre, was at that time nowhere in the picture. Catherine de' Medici, going from Florence to France to marry the future King Henry II, took her own perfumer with her, to keep her in the scented manner to which she was accustomed. (He opened a shop in Paris under the name of René.) One of the fashions in Italy was the wearing of scented gloves, and the Earl of Oxford, after a visit to Italy, introduced the craze into the English court. The queen herself had several pairs and was girlishly proud of them.

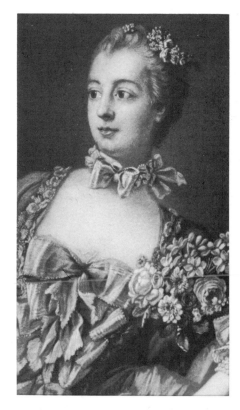

Elizabeth was fascinated by perfumes of all kinds. We know two of her favourite scents. One was made of musk and roses: 'Take 8 grains of musk and put in rose water 8 spoonfuls, 3 spoonfuls of damask water, and a quarter of an ounce of sugar. Boil for five hours and strain it'. The damask water was an extract of damask roses; the sugar was probably a preservative. Another of Elizabeth's perfumes has a more mysterious recipe: 'Take 8 spoonfuls of compound water, the weight of twopence in fine powder of sugar, and boil it on hot embers and coals softly, add half an ounce of sweet marjoram dried in the sun, and the weight of twopence of the powder of benjamin'. And what was compound water? We do not know.

The queen spent extravagantly on perfumes. In 1584 she paid £40 in wages to her 'stillers of sweet waters', John Kraunckwell and his wife – enough to keep them in solid middle-class comfort. Another of her perfumers was Ralph Rabbards, who made up a number of special waters for her. He once wrote to her offering his 'odours moste sweet and delicate' and recommending especially water of violets and gillyflower water. This early example of selling by direct mail also offered waters 'to cleanse and keep bright the skynne and flesh and to preserve it in a perfect state.'

It all sounds very idyllic – 'sweet' flower waters, odours 'moste delicate'. We have to make an effort of imagination to appreciate that the scents of Elizabeth's court would have been far too pungent for our modern noses. They had to overcome the stench of unwashed bodies and unwashed clothes. Hungary water was still popular, but musk and civet were the basis of most scents. Still, it does seem that Elizabeth's tastes were more subtle than those of most of the ladies of her court.

Not only in England were the perfumes of the day horrifyingly potent. In 1580 one of the earliest popular books on cosmetics was published in France. *Les secrets de Maistre Alexys le Piedmontois* advocated a toilet water that it claimed would make women 'beautiful for ever'. The recipe is frightening: 'take a young raven from its nest, feed it on hard-boiled eggs for forty days, kill it, then distill it with myrtle leaves, talcum powder, and almond oil'.

The mixture owed more to magic than to cosmetic science. This sort of alchemical recipe continued to be used until well into the 18th century, side by side with pungent-smelling products designed more to swamp the stench of unwashed womanhood than to enhance female sex appeal. The change to modern habits happened in France.

Madame de Pompadour, mistress of Louis XV, lavished perfume on herself on a scale that makes Queen Elizabeth seem a beginner. But Madame de Pompadour was a lover of flowers, and of scented flowers in particular, and she went in for more delicate fragrances and more 'natural' scents than had previously been the

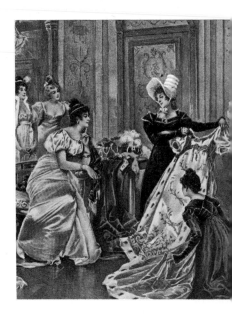

Above: the Empress Josephine chooses a new gown. Already a leader of Parisian society when Napoleon married her in 1796, Josephine enjoyed fine clothes, cosmetics, and perfumes. Like Madame de Pompadour, she was fond of hyacinths and grew them as pot plants in her rooms. She also liked mignonette – perhaps because its scent is rather like that of the violet. Napoleon took time out from his Egyptian campaign to send some mignonette seed home to her. Mignonette became a popular button-hole flower for Parisian society and it became fashionable also to grow the plant on verandahs and balconies — its perfume being so strong that it masked the odours from the streets.

fashion. She was the pioneer. Marie Antoinette, Louis XVI's queen, followed the same path and set Europe firmly on the perfumed road it has followed ever since. Marie Antoinette disliked spicy eastern perfumes and heavy animal scents and established a fashion for lighter, pleasanter perfumes distilled from roses and violets. She also popularized again the pleasures of the bath, which Europe had almost forgotten since the fall of Rome. Her example made the fragrant bath once again an important part of a lady's toilet. Some of her ladies went further than their mistress. One of them, Madame Tallier, used to bathe in crushed strawberries whenever they were in season – which may have been pleasing to the nose but must have been fairly repulsive to the eye. Madame Tallier was also a latter-day Poppaea; she washed in perfumed milk.

The change in fashion survived the upheaval of the French revolution. Napoleon's wife Josephine followed Marie Antoinette's tastes and preferred simple, natural scents. She had a passion for violets and liked jasmine – unless Napoleon, who once gave her a present of a bottle of jasmine, made a husbandly mistake and presented her with a gift she didn't want. But Josephine was a creole, brought up in Martinique where the natives made oils and creams of almond and coconut, and perhaps she merely pretended to conform to the more insipid European taste. We know that she was fond of musk and that she bought several lots of almond cream from her Parisian perfumer. Or perhaps she was simply trying to please Napoleon. He was fussy about what scent she wore, and it has been said that the only perfumes he would allow her to use in his presence were orange water, lavender water, and eau de Cologne.

Eau de Cologne was a new scent in Josephine's time. At the beginning of the 18th century, Paul Feminis, an Italian living in the German city of Cologne, had brought out a toilet water that at last pushed Hungary water into second place on the sales charts. It was based on citrus oils, neroli, lemon, bergamot, and lavender. Under the name of *l'eau admirable* it lasted for almost a hundred years. Then Jean Marie Farina, a descendant of Feminis, altered the formula slightly, incorporating rosemary into it, and marketed the new product under the name *eau de Cologne*. It was an immediate runaway success, was copied by many other perfumers, and began a fashion for gentle toilet waters that has lasted until our own day. In Paris, Pierre Guerlain produced a water with a lavender base. Guerlain had friends at the court of Napoleon III. They introduced it to the empress Eugenie. She loved it and recommended it to Parisian society. It made the name of Guerlain famous throughout Europe and was named, in honour of Eugenie, eau de Cologne Imperiale.

The 19th century was the great age of toilet waters. It was also a very boring age in terms of perfume – Marie Antoinette had done her work too well. It was

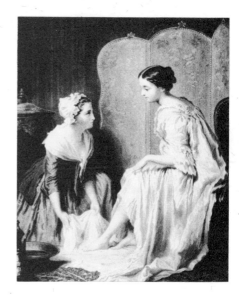

Above and below: two views of the divide between upstairs and downstairs in Victorian England. The maid giving a foot-bath to her young mistress would not have been allowed to wear an obtrusive perfume while in the presence of her employer – although in her off-duty hours she might use some of the potent, cheap perfumes that were beginning to be sold in the shops. Her mistress would have been scented only delicately with a mild and respectable toilet water, but the maid was not expected to imitate her betters – as the cartoon *below* makes clear.

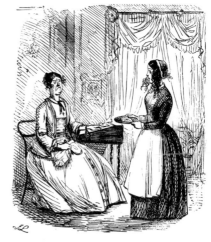

AN IMPUDENT MINX.

Lady of the House. "HOITY TOITY, INDEED? GO AND PUT UP THOSE CURLS DIRECTLY, IF YOU PLEASE. HOW DARE YOU IMITATE ME IN THAT MANNER? IMPERTINENCE!"

perhaps the first century that would not have offended our own sense of smell. Women were cleaner, and they smelled pleasantly enough. But compared with what had gone before they were insipidly perfumed. Strong perfumes were mostly cheap perfumes, and were left to shop-girls and tarts. Respectable women smelled of such things as lavender and rosemary, and they used perfume meanly. There might be lavender sachets in the clothes closets, and in country houses the daughters of the family might make dainty pot-pourri. But the days of the lavish, imaginative, and sexy use of perfumes were over. Past ages had drenched their bodies and their hair in scent. They had scattered it over their floors, burned it in their rooms. They had worn scented gloves and scented clothes. They had bathed in perfume. They had worn rings that ejected spurts of scent on to their lovers as they bent to kiss their hands. They had pressed their lovers' lips to scented nipples, cupped liquid perfume in their navels. All this was forgotten. At a time when manufacturing perfumers were beginning to produce in industrial quantities the greatest variety of attractive scents that the world had known, the women of Europe could think of no other use for perfume than to place two drops of it behind their ears.

Below: 'I prefer it to any other.' An 188? advertisement for Pears' soap relied on the unemphatic recommendation of Lillie Langtry — actress, society beauty, and mistress of the Prince of Wales. Other Pears' advertisements of about the same time make modest mention of the soap's 'agreeable and lasting perfume' and claim that its use guarantees a 'good complexion and nice hands'. Cosmetics and perfumes at this stage were still suspect; unobtrusiveness was the ideal.

Right: a perfume advertisement of the 1970s uses modern techniques of persuasion to stress the exotic allure of a sophisticated modern perfume.

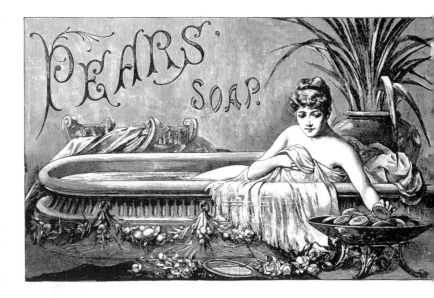

Only as we draw towards the end of the 20th century has perfume shown signs of coming once again into its own. The young of the 1970s are beginning to use simpler, stronger scents and to use them more imaginatively. They burn sticks of incense, light perfumed candles. And, recovering at last from Victorian hang-ups over sex, they are beginning to rediscover the erotic attraction of perfume on their bodies.

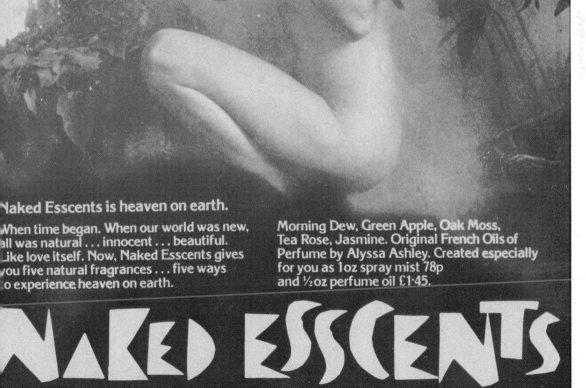

Naked Esscents is heaven on earth.

When time began. When our world was new,
all was natural . . . innocent . . . beautiful.
Like love itself. Now, Naked Esscents gives
you five natural fragrances . . . five ways
to experience heaven on earth.

Morning Dew, Green Apple, Oak Moss,
Tea Rose, Jasmine. Original French Oils of
Perfume by Alyssa Ashley. Created especially
for you as 1oz spray mist 78p
and ½oz perfume oil £1·45.

NaKed ESSCeNTS

Napoleon was fond of violets only because Josephine liked them. But violets survived the divorce and death of Josephine and became part of the Napoleonic legend. In this print — an English copy of one distributed in Paris after Napoleon's return from Elba — it is his second wife, Maria Louisa of Austria, who faces him in the hidden profiles formed by the flowers and whose son is pictured beneath his parents.

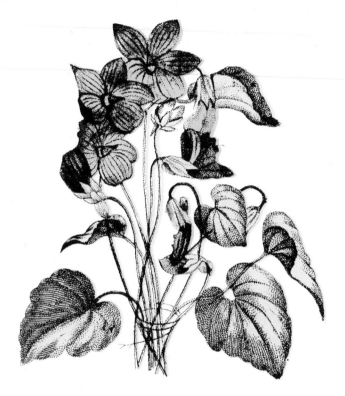

CORPORAL VIOLET,

Buonaparte having on his departure for the Island of Elba, promised his Confidential Friends to return in the Violet Season, his adherents adopted the above simple Flower as a Rallying Signal. "CORPORAL VIOLET" became their favorite Toast, and each was distinguished by a Gold Ring with a Violet in Enamel, and the motto "Elle reparaitra au printems!" (It will appear again in spring.) As soon as it became generally known that he had Landed at Frejus, a multitude of the Women of Paris were seen with Baskets full of these Flowers, which were purchased and worn by His Friends, without exciting the least suspicion. It was customary on meeting any one thus decorated, to ask "Aimez vouz-la violette?" (Do you like the Violet?) when if they answered 'Oui'. (Yes.) it was certain the party was not a confederate. But if the reply was 'Eh bien'. (Well.) they recognised an adherent, and completed the sentence "Elle reparaitra au printems!" The original Print of which the above is a correct Copy, was also published at Paris, with the same symbolical meaning; in which may be traced the Profiles of Buonaparte and Maria Louisa, watching over their Infant Child.

Today only the conservative middle-aged cling to the feeling that perfumes are effeminate. But it is in fact only in the last two decades that it has become possible for a man to be scented without being thought unmanly. Right up to the years after World War II men were supposed to smell only of tobacco, tweed, and beer, but not – although some women claim to be turned on by it – of male sweat.

That men today are scented with pre- and after-shave lotions, with body-splash colognes, with talcum powders, and with hair sprays is not in the least strange. It is far stranger that the habit was ever lost. At most periods in history perfume has been a unisex thing. Men have usually been as highly scented as women, and sometimes more highly scented.

The obvious analogy with the scented male is the long-haired male. Long hair for men has been the norm rather than the exception. Only for relatively short periods, on the historical time scale, have men been short-haired. But one of those periods happened to coincide more or less with late Victorian and Edwardian times in Britain. It was the same with perfume. Men have nearly always been perfumed, but the Victorians gave us a hang-up about it that deeply inhibited the male use of scent. It took two world wars to break down the barriers and make men scented again.

Even so, we still haven't completely recovered. We still use perfume with what to most societies at most times would have seemed unimaginative restraint. A Western man going out to dinner today would, if he thought of scents at all, think only of the scent of food. But he would confidently expect to be offered a drink. Yet, had he lived in, for example, ancient Egypt, he would equally confidently have expected to be offered a choice of perfume. What would happen?

As soon as the guest arrived, a slave would anoint his head with perfume. Another would garland his neck with lotus flowers. He would perhaps be presented with a cone of aromatic wax to place upon his head. As the evening wore on the wax would melt and run down on to his neck and shoulders, coating him with fragrance. In the banqueting hall itself floral wreaths would be hung upon the walls, and tables and floor would be strewn with scented flowers.

None of this was for the benefit of women guests, like the flowers on the table for ladies' night at the Rotary

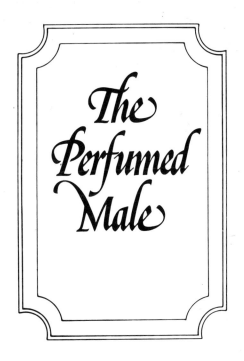

The Perfumed Male

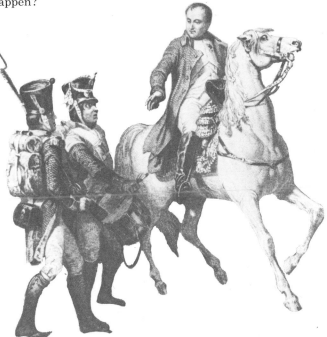

Napoleon's favourite perfume was eau de Cologne, which he used extravagantly throughout his life. Even on campaign – *below*, crossing the Elbe, 1813 – he would pour it over his neck and shoulders every time he washed.

Club. Scents were part of the luxurious sensuous environment that surrounded any rich Egyptian. Indeed, Egyptian men may well have used perfumes before Egyptian women. They had a tradition that seems to date right back to the neolithic period – when the peoples who were to form the Egyptian nation were still hunters and herdsmen in the Nile valley – of their ancestors smearing their bodies with scented grease and oil from the castor plant. Civilized Egyptians doubtless looked back upon these greasy forebears with the same half-superior, half-respectful feelings that we have towards the woad-painted ancient Britons. But they kept the habit up, and used scent with a liberality that is hard for us to imagine.

When, in 361 B.C., Agesilaus, king of Sparta, came to Egypt and was entertained at a banquet with all the scented trimmings, he thought it all so decadent and effeminate that he refused to have any part of it and stalked away in disgust. His astonished hosts merely thought him totally uncivilized and uncouth. It is a neat example of two opposing attitudes to the male use of scents.

We must not make Agesilaus' mistake. There was nothing effeminate about the men of ancient Egypt, or of the other great nations of the ancient Middle East. But these were probably the most lavish splashers-around of perfume in the whole of recorded history. The Mycenaeans, who were as cleanly a people as the Egyptians, covered themselves with a variety of perfumed oils and unguents. Mycenaean men used ornate alabaster toilet jars to hold ointments made by boiling together coriander, ginger grass, wine, and honey. The kings of Persia wore crowns made of myrrh and of a scented plant called labyzus. In their palaces incense was constantly kept burning in ornate and richly decorated censers. When one of the greatest of their kings, Darius, was defeated by Alexander the Great at the battle of Arbela, he abandoned in his tent all the treasures he had taken with him on campaign. They included a casket filled with precious aromatics. Alexander, reacting as Agesilaus had done, had the casket thrown out in disgust.

The man who was perhaps the biggest spender at the perfumer's of all time was Antiochus IV, king of Syria from 175 to 164 B.C. At the games he organized at Daphne, not far from Antioch, a procession of two hundred glamorous women, each carrying a golden bowl of perfume, sprinkled the watchers with costly and exquisite scents. The thousands of special guests who received VIP treatment were anointed on their arrival with the perfume of their choice from a selection including saffron, cinnamon, spikenard, and lilies. As a parting gift, when the long-drawn-out celebrations ended, each received a crown of myrrh and frankincense.

Only rarely do we have candid-camera cameos of any of the great rulers of the ancient world, but it so happens

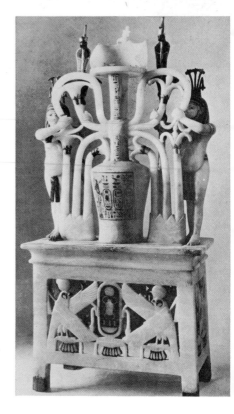

Above: one of the ornate perfume vases found in the tomb of Tutankhamun. Perfume accompanied every Egyptian pharaoh throughout his life and remained with him in his tomb. Or that, at least, was the intention. Perfumes rarely stayed in the tombs for long – they were as attractive to robbers as precious stones are to thieves today. Tutankhamun's tomb – one of the smallest in the Valley of Kings – was missed by robbers because its entrance was buried under the rubble from the building of another tomb. Its vases of unguents remained untouched until the burial chamber was entered in 1922. When they were opened they released the scent that had been sealed in 3,000 years before – the scent of spikenard. The unguents had solidified into a sticky mass of yellow lumps in a chocolate-coloured body, but enough remained to analyse. Ninety per cent was animal fat; the remaining 10 per cent was a mixture of gum resins and 'something resembling Indian spikenard'.

that we have one of Antiochus. He was once relaxing in the public baths when a man came up to him and said, 'You must be a happy man. You smell most richly'. Antiochus, perhaps secretly pleased and flattered, but wanting to punish the man for his temerity in so unceremoniously approaching a king, played an expensive practical joke. He ordered his attendants to pour a huge ewerful of unguent over the man's head. Much of it dripped to the floor from the man's drenched body, and a crowd collected to gather up these valuable slops. The sight made Antiochus laugh. But he laughed so much that he slipped in the pool of unguent and sat down suddenly and unregally. This, in the staid phrase of Eugene Rimmel, 'put an end to his merriment'.

Middle-eastern potentates like Antiochus were the tutors in perfumery to the world. From them Greek men caught the perfume habit and became sometimes more scented than their women. As early as Homeric times it was a Greek custom to offer arriving guests a bath and to anoint them with aromatic oils before they sat down to eat. By the time of Xenophanes, around the turn of the sixth and fifth centuries B.C., Greek banquets rivalled those of Egypt in their scented extravagance:

> *each guest upon his forehead bears*
> *A wreathed, flowery crown; from slender vase*
> *A willing youth presents to each in turn*
> *A sweet and costly perfume . . .*
> *While odorous gums fill all the room.*

At one banquet, doves whose wings had been saturated with a variety of perfumes were released to fly around the room. At others, scented oils and wines streamed from one or other of the bodily orifices of statues. The guests themselves were individually highly scented. The fashion of applying different perfumes to different parts of the body was a unisex one, followed by men as well as women:

> *His jaws and breasts he rubs with thick palm oil,*
> *And both his arms with extract sweet of mint;*
> *His eyebrows and his hair with marjoram,*
> *His knees and neck with essence of ground thyme.*

Not everyone, of course, went along with the fashion. The cynic philosopher Diogenes took a severely practical attitude to the application of scent. He used perfumes, but only on his feet, explaining that the smell then rose up to his nose, while if he anointed the upper part of his body the scent was lost in the air and benefitted only the birds. Theophrastus suggests that, in any case, Greek men of his day tended to wear lighter perfumes than their women and, perhaps, used it with rather more restraint. He mentions a solid perfume that was crumbled into powder and sprinkled on to the bed, so that it rubbed off on the sleeper's body during the night. 'In this way the perfume gets a better hold and is more lasting. Men use it thus, instead of scenting their bodies directly.'

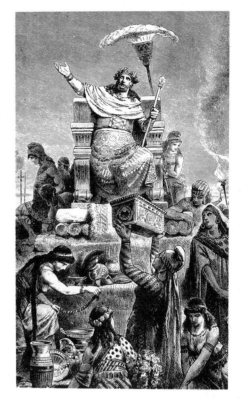

Above: the prospect of a scented death for Croesus, king of Lydia. There are several versions of the Croesus story. One tale has it that, defeated by the Persian king Cyrus in 546 B.C., Croesus decided to go out in a blaze of glory. He had his personal treasures piled against a huge pyre of fragrant woods and gums. He clambered to a throne on top of the pyre, ordered the torch to be applied, and awaited death in the flames. His gesture was spoilt when a torrential downpour inconsiderately put out the blaze. Another version of the story is that Cyrus condemned Croesus to be burned to death, but pardoned him at the last moment. Both accounts agree that Croesus lived on and became a trusted adviser to his ex-enemy Cyrus. Legend allows another king, Ashurbanipal of Assyria, a more successful suicide on a scented bonfire. Eighty years before Croesus, Ashurbanipal, together with his wives, died of asphyxiation in the sweet, perfumed fumes of a similar pyre.

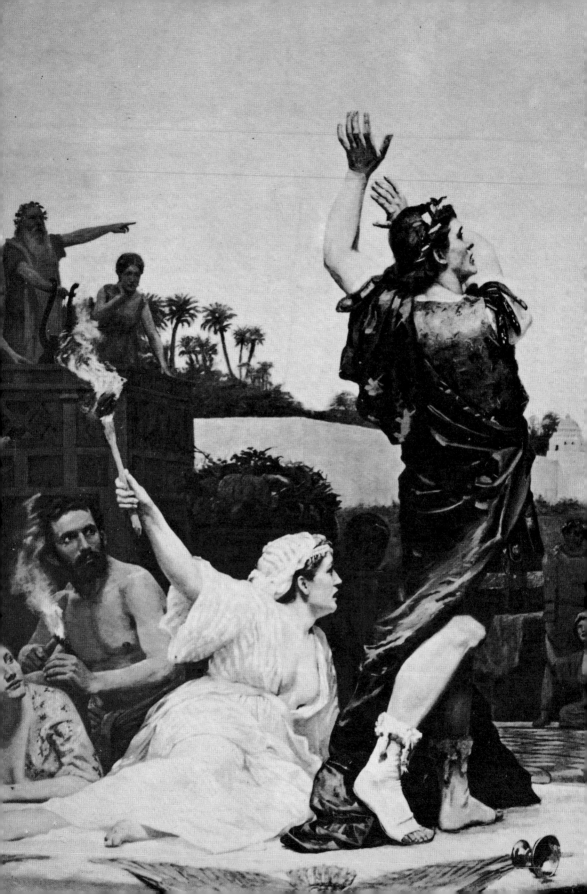

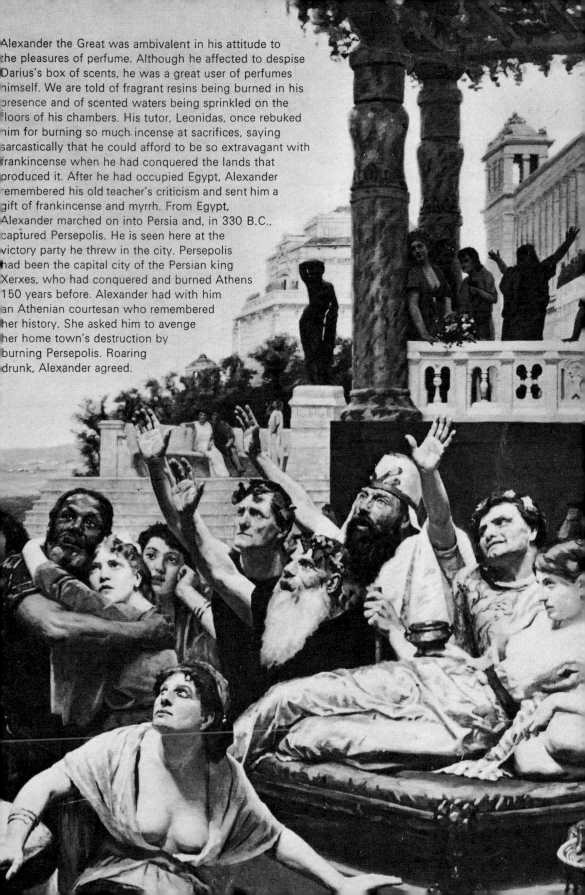

Alexander the Great was ambivalent in his attitude to the pleasures of perfume. Although he affected to despise Darius's box of scents, he was a great user of perfumes himself. We are told of fragrant resins being burned in his presence and of scented waters being sprinkled on the floors of his chambers. His tutor, Leonidas, once rebuked him for burning so much incense at sacrifices, saying sarcastically that he could afford to be so extravagant with frankincense when he had conquered the lands that produced it. After he had occupied Egypt, Alexander remembered his old teacher's criticism and sent him a gift of frankincense and myrrh. From Egypt, Alexander marched on into Persia and, in 330 B.C., captured Persepolis. He is seen here at the victory party he threw in the city. Persepolis had been the capital city of the Persian king Xerxes, who had conquered and burned Athens 150 years before. Alexander had with him an Athenian courtesan who remembered her history. She asked him to avenge her home town's destruction by burning Persepolis. Roaring drunk, Alexander agreed.

Since the Greeks' sexual habits are well-known, it should perhaps be pointed out that a man's love for boys is homosexual and not effeminate and that the Greeks, in any case, were not homosexual but ambisexual. The Greek male's love of perfume does not, therefore, provide ammunition to those who still think perfume unmanly. If that were so, Roman men – who went in for straight sex with undertones of sadism – would not so eagerly have copied the Greeks. Roman men, too, anointed their whole bodies with aromatic oils; it was an important part of the ritual of the Roman bath – which, we have to remember, was largely a male preserve. Rich Romans soaked their clothing in scents. Some even rubbed their pets and horses with perfumed oils – so that the master came not only to look like his dog but to smell like it. Roman soldiers returning from campaigns in the East brought back with them – as did the Crusaders later – male cosmetics and mysterious, heavy perfumes that had come to them by way of India. At least one Roman lived to regret his fondness for perfume. Lucius Plotius, sought by the authorities because he was the brother of a consul who had been proscribed, fled from Rome and went into hiding in Salerno. He was discovered, according to Pliny, because he used a perfume so strong and distinctive that it led his hunters to his hiding place.

As we might expect, it was some of the big spenders among the Roman emperors who were most lavish with scents. Caligula spent enormous sums on scented ointments and was a great believer in the efficacy of scented baths to restore a body jaded by sexual excesses. Nero cherished the same belief. He surrounded himself with scents. At Poppaea's funeral – she was embalmed like an Egyptian queen – it is said that the incense Nero ordered to be burned was the equivalent of a whole year's supply from Arabia. In his great palace in Rome, the Golden House, Nero had dining rooms built with ceilings of fretted ivory. Concealed pipes sprayed perfume down on to his guests and panels slid aside to shower them with scented flower blossoms. It has also been reported that every room in the Golden House was carpeted several inches deep with red rose petals – but this was probably only on special occasions. Otho, the next-but-one emperor, had been a friend of Nero and a lover of Poppaea, and he shared with them both a liking for perfumes. When he went on a military campaign he took with him a whole range of scents as well as cosmetics. In this he differed from another, greater, Roman soldier. Julius Caesar belonged to the anti-scent school. He once said to a particularly highly scented fop, 'I'd rather you stank of garlic'.

The tradition of the bathed and perfumed male disappeared from Europe as the Romans withdrew. The Europe of the Dark Ages threw away all that was good in Roman civilization along with all that it thought to be

Right: another of Sir Lawrence Alma-Tadema's highly romanticized pictures of ancient life – this time a scene in a Roman bath. In fact women rarely used the public baths. They were social and leisure centres mainly for men, who went to them as they might go to the golf club today. All had hot and cold baths and anointing and massage parlours. Some of the larger ones had also public rooms for drink and conversation, picture galleries, libraries, and gymnasiums for exercise. Caracalla's baths, on the outskirts of Rome, could seat – on polished marble – more than two thousand bathers at a time.

Socrates (*below*) was one of those Greeks who disapproved of men using perfume. Free men, he pronounced crushingly, should smell only of 'free labours and manly exercise'.

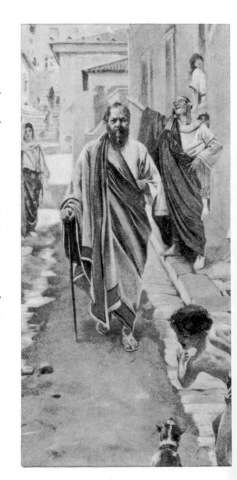

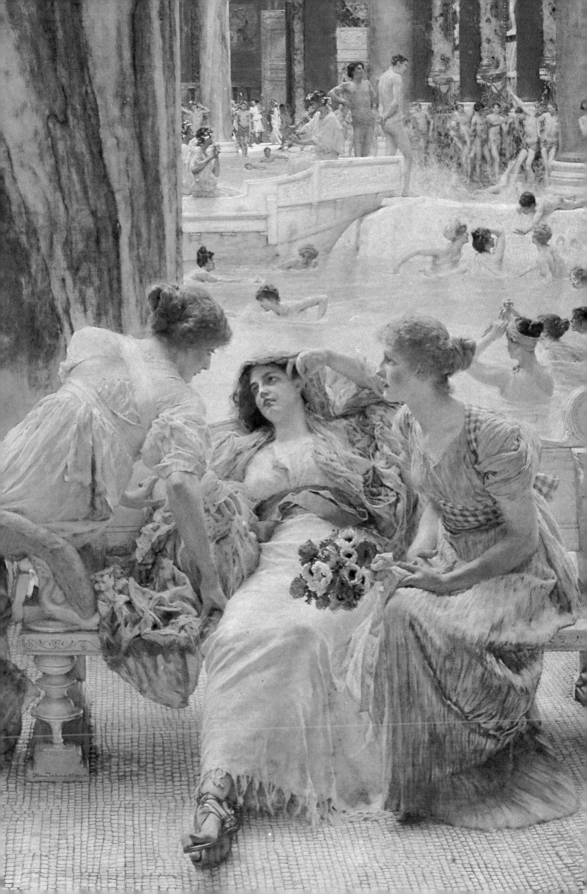

bad. The thinking was simple. The Romans washed, had sanitation, were perfumed, and made love. The Roman empire had fallen. Why? Clearly, because the Romans washed, had sanitation, were perfumed, and made love. All this was obviously cause and effect, and could be summed up in the one word 'decadence'. Decadence was therefore to be avoided at all costs. Happily throwing away the Roman baby with the Roman bathwater, Europe turned its back firmly on the luxuries of Rome. Among these, of course, was perfume. Christianity, too, helped to push the reactionary band-wagon, both because of its antagonism to all things Roman as a result of memories of the persecutions, and because the early Christian Fathers were frightened of self-indulgence. The Church added its weight to the anti-washing, anti-perfume forces.

The Arabs kept the flag of perfume flying during Europe's Dark Ages. It was a rose red flag. Rose water was the Arabs' favourite scent, as it was to become the Europeans'. Legend has it that some of the caliphs had fountains of rose water playing in their palaces. One of them, El-Mutawkkel, had the rugs in all his apartments

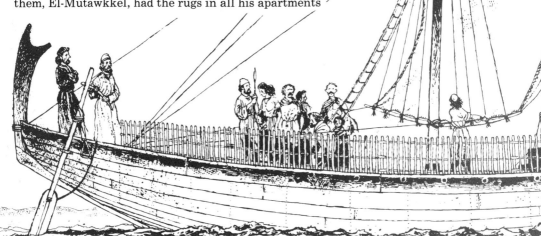

continually sprinkled with rose water and declared 'I am the king of all sultans, as the rose is the king of all fragrances'. Saladin, as soon as he entered Jerusalem in 1187, ordered the floors and walls of Omar's Mosque to be thoroughly washed down with rose water.

There were glimmers of light even in Europe. A few courts, and a few eccentrics, continued to use scents and the idea once again caught on. One of the pioneers of the Western resurgence was the emperor Charlemagne. Soon after his coronation in A.D. 800, he received from the Caliph Harun al-Raschid in Baghdad a present of the most costly perfumes and a white elephant. But it was the Crusades that really brought scent back to the men of Europe.

The Crusades came as a traumatic shock to western European men. They came into contact with peoples whose customs and habits were totally different from

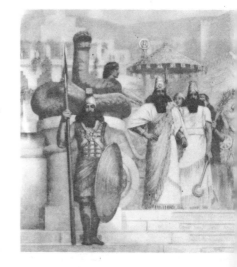

their own cherished ones, yet whose civilization was clearly highly successful. These infidels – although they were routinely condemned by the propaganda machines of the day as savage and cruel and, indeed, decadent – were clearly neither weak nor effete. They kept winning battles. And many returning knights bore the scars that proved they had met better men than themselves – better, cleaner, more scented men.

The Crusaders were tempted, and fell. They brought back, as we have seen, exotic perfumes for their women. They brought back rose water for themselves. They also brought back the idea of the bath. In their home towns in Europe they set up public baths that were copies of those they had seen in the Levant. 'By the 13th century', says Maggie Angeloglou in *A history of make-up*, 'these public baths were being used regularly by townspeople, and in some areas a recollection of Rome returned, for sweating rooms were added in which eminent citizens would meet to discuss business and local affairs.' The Church authorities objected. In France at least they succeeded in closing down most of the baths. England held on, sporadically, until Tudor times.

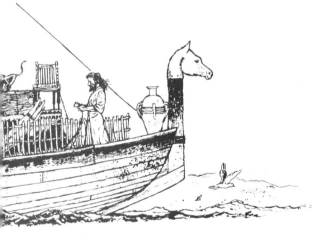

The story of bathing and of personal cleanliness is important to our own story. We can make a series of wild generalizations about cleanliness and the male use of scent. The men of the ancient world were clean and scented. European men of the Dark Ages were dirty and unscented. Those of medieval times, and of modern times up to about the end of the 17th century, were dirty and scented. Eighteenth-century men were clean and scented. Nineteenth-century men were clean and unscented. We have, of course, to make many modifications and reservations about this sweeping series of accusations, but it is a useful yardstick to hold in mind while remembering that there is a great difference between perfumes used to conceal or swamp the smell of the unwashed body and those that, starting as it were with a clean sheet, are intended to impart a newly attractive odour to the human body.

Left: a Phoenician merchant ship carrying a cargo of slaves, spices, and incense. Over the centuries the Phoenicians played a greater part than any other peoples in the development of the scent trade. With prosperous colonies all round the Mediterranean, they were the shippers of the ancient world. Almost every cargo that was carried by sea was despatched if not in Phoenician vessels then in ships built by them for other powers. Egypt, Assyria, and Persia all had fleets of the up-to-date cedarwood ships built by the Phoenician shipyards. With their nearest rivals, the Greeks, the Phoenicians shared a near-monopoly of the seas, and they grew rich and powerful by shipping, in particular, the raw materials for incense and perfume production. Their political expertise enabled them to hang on – sometimes only by their fingertips – to control of their most important natural asset, the cedarwood forests of Lebanon. They had a monopoly also of the purple dye extracted from the shellfish murex – a dye so precious in the ancient world that purple became the symbolic colour of royalty.

Below left: Babylonian and Assyrian men were as highly perfumed as their women. To our eyes, they would have looked very effeminate. They wore jewelry and heavy make-up and their beards – to them, symbols of manhood – were glued into intricate curls and ringlets with perfumed setting lotions. Ashurbanipal, last of the kings of Assyria, was – if we are to judge from some of the activities depicted on the walls of his palace at Nineveh – a thoroughly masculine man in everything that mattered. But he wore rouge and eye paint and sometimes dressed in women's clothes; they were, he said, more attractive than men's. According to one story – another we have already seen (p. 93) – Ashurbanipal's effeminate habits caused his death. One of his generals, by name Arbaces, walked in on the king one day and caught him in the act of pencilling his eyebrows. Arbaces was so disgusted by the sight that he drew his dagger and stabbed Ashurbanipal to death on the spot.

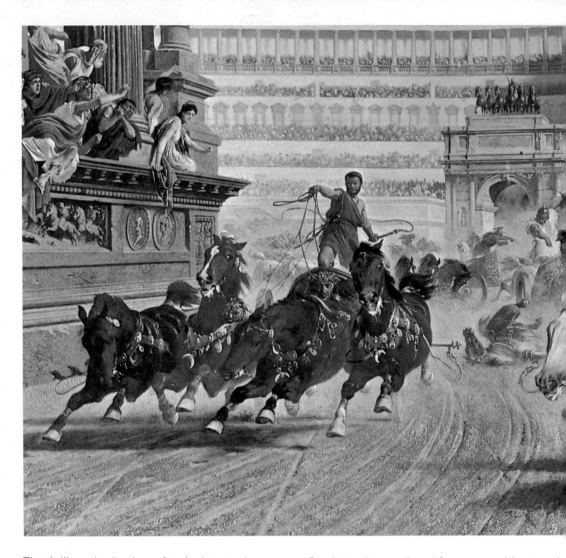

The thrills and splendour of a chariot race in a
Roman arena, reconstructed — with considerable
accuracy — by the 19th-century painter
Alexander Wagner. Around the 'royal box' where
the emperor sits are lamps burning fragrant gums.
Huge awnings — which were sometimes
drenched in perfume — shade some of the
spectators sweltering in the crowded tiers of
seats. (The emperor Caligula — whose jokes were
usually cruel — enjoyed having these awnings
removed at the hottest time of day and
forbidding any of the spectators to leave.)
Enormous crowds attended the chariot races —
the great Circus Maximus in Rome could seat
260,000 people. A day out at the circus was to
the Roman holiday-maker rather like Derby Day
to us — but more congested, more splendid, more
ceremonious, and more thrilling. There was
always the chance, or hope, of a gory accident.

Chariot racing produced far more accidents and
far more fatalities than motor racing today. The
'games' in the Roman arenas were, of course,
immeasurably worse. There the stench of blood
and death from the sand-strewn arena added to
the living smell from the hot, crowded, excited
spectators. A colosseum opened in Rome in
A.D. 80 had seating for 45,000 spectators and
standing room for another 5,000 — all crammed
tightly together in the heat. The smell must have
been appalling. Stalls and itinerant salesmen did
a thriving trade selling cooling, perfumed
unguents to the crowds who had come to watch
certain death and certain torture. Gladiatorial
combats between two, four, or six fighters were
only the overture to large-scale massacres.
Criminals of both sexes and all ages were
dragged into the arena to be torn to bloody
death by wild animals. Full-scale battles were

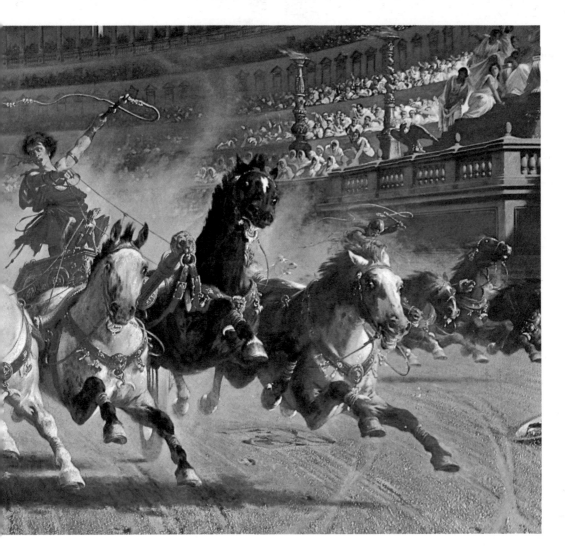

staged. The emperor Agrippa once enjoyed a
battle, fought to the death, between two armies
of 700 men. He was a merciful man compared to
Trajan, who, in one period of four months, sent
10,000 gladiators to fight in the arena. Most
spectacular of all were the sea battles. The arena
was flooded — or sometimes lakes were
specially dug — and fleets of ships, manned by
condemned criminals, battled until the water
crimsoned with blood. Three thousand men
fought in one 'naval engagement' organized by
Julius Caesar. One or two emperors, less sadistic
than the rest, tried to replace this butchery by
games in the Greek style. Greek games (*right*)
were trials of skill and strength between equals.
Competitors fought, not for their lives, but for the
victor's trophy in the shape of a golden violet --
the scented flower that became the symbol of
the ancient city of Athens.

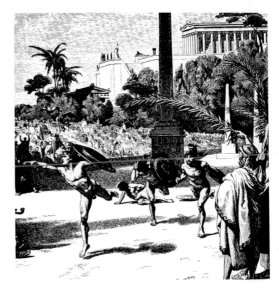

The Tudors certainly had no fine feelings about cleanliness, but by their time scents had become very much part of the everyday life of the wealthy and middle classes. Rose water was still the most popular scent. Men used it to sprinkle over their heads and their clothes and, less often, their bodies – which rarely saw the light of day. In John Marston's play, *The History of Antonio and Mellida,* performed in 1602, one character is a young gallant who sprinkles perfume over himself from a casting bottle – a porcelain bottle with holes in the top like a sugar caster. We have a contemporary recipe for scent to fill a casting bottle. It is rose water to which is added small quantities of spikenard, thyme, lemon, cloves, and a touch of civet.

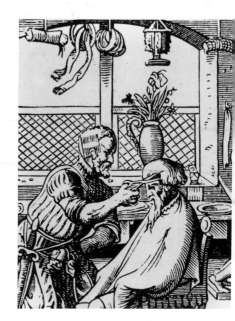

Rose water, and other floral waters, were also sprinkled on to Tudor floors. So were rushes and other plants that released their scent when crushed underfoot. Men carried pomanders. Scented gloves were worn by men as well as women. In the houses of the rich, silver bowls filled with rose water were placed in the bedrooms and clothes were kept in chests made of scented woods such as juniper, cedar, and sandalwood. Full-time servants were employed to fumigate and perfume the rooms of great houses. There were also itinerant perfumers and fumigators, 'selling rotten wood by the pound . . . which gentlemen burn by the ounce', according to Beaumont and Fletcher's play *Wit Without Money*. No one thought any of this unmanly.

The Tudors were following a perfumed fashion set by the European courts of the 15th century and in particular, as we saw in the previous chapter, by Italy. The French courts too had been scented. Henry III was a great scent user and under his influence even wholly masculine men – which the king was not – were scented and painted.

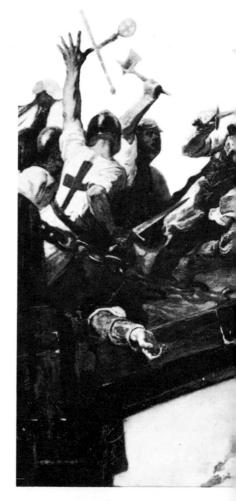

In England, however, the Puritans put an end to scented extravagance, which did not return until the Restoration. Under Charles II gentlemen once again took to using scented waters. Over in France, Louis XIV had pages whose job it was to see that the air of the state apartments was always perfumed with rose water and marjoram. Louis was called in his own day 'the sweetest-scented monarch' the world had ever seen. His shirts were always rinsed in his own special perfumed water, which was made by simmering aloes, nutmeg, cloves, storax, and benzoin in rose-water for twenty-four hours and then adding jasmine and orange water and a few grains of musk.

The 17th century also saw the return to favour of the bath. In London, Duke's Bagnio and Bath opened in 1679. It was quickly followed by a number of competitors – 'sweating houses' that offered Turkish baths, mineral baths, and perfumed baths. This was the result of a new feeling, partially a result of the plague years, that cleanliness was important after all. The bath

Left: a contemporary wood-engraving of a 16th-century barber's shop. Only a wealthy dandy would have his hair shampooed — the age was not one in which the ordinary man made a fetish of cleanliness. The vase at the window is filled with flowers and herbs whose scent combatted that of unwashed clothes — the barber's slashed and padded jacket is typical of the thick clothes that made the Elizabethans so smelly. *Below:* the Crusaders take Jerusalem. In bloody battles such as this the Crusaders were forced to realize that the scent-loving Mahomedans were not effeminate weaklings but tough and savage fighting men.

The Roman emperor Heliogabalus was as extravagant a voluptuary as Nero and the scented scene *overleaf* is little exaggerated. The huge censer of burning incense, the emperor's coronet of flowers, and the cascade of rose petals swamping his courtiers — all are well authenticated. Heliogabalus had been brought up in Syria and had absorbed eastern tastes and habits — mainly those of eastern women. He made his triumphal entry into Rome in A.D. 218 in a preposterous sort of drag. He wore enormous ear rings, his eyes were painted with concentric rings of blue and gold, his lips were gilded, and his hands and feet dyed with henna.

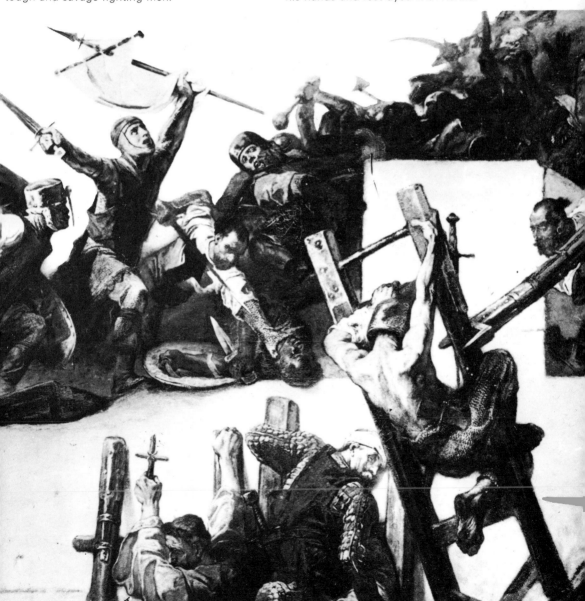

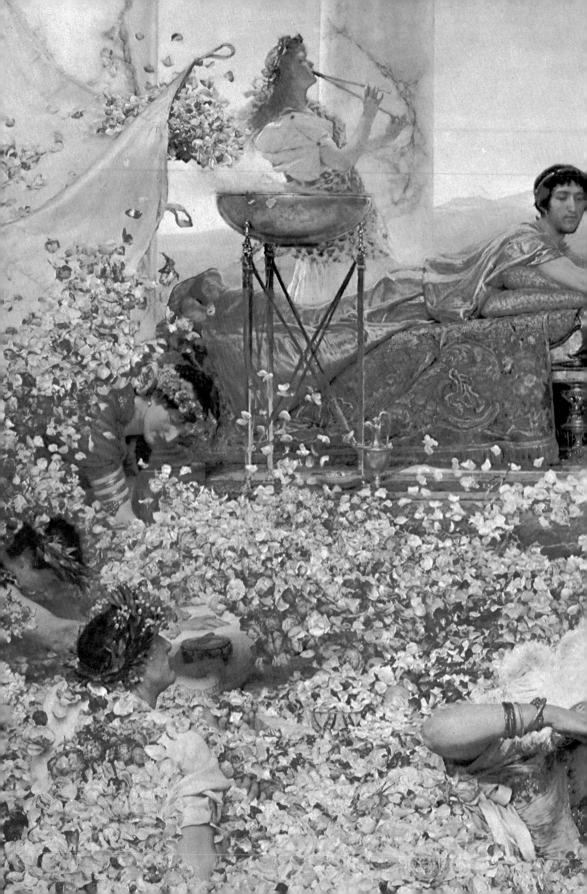

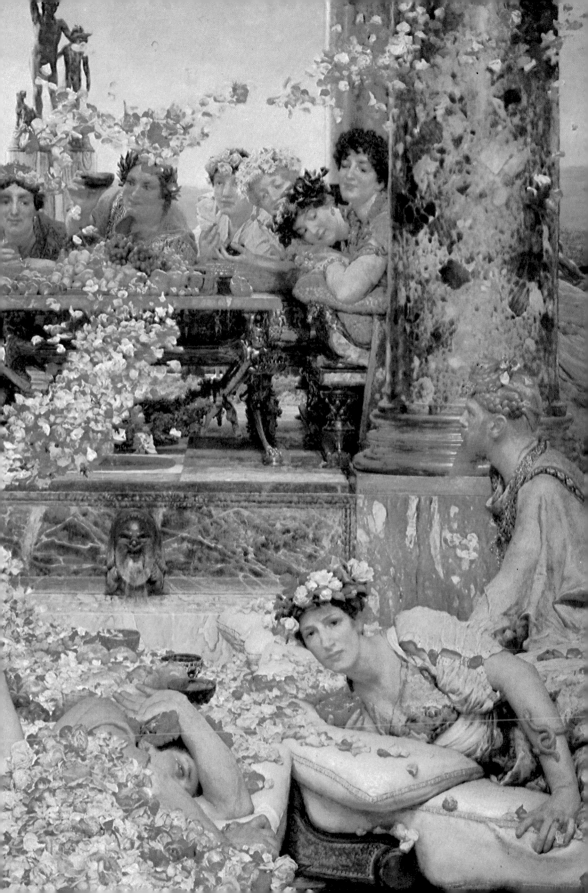

again became a sybaritic pleasure. Soaps – as well as perfumes – were beyond the purses of most men, as indeed they always had been, but young men about town began to take a foppish pride in personal cleanliness. By 1765 the young gallant in London could go to Hummums in Covent Garden and, for an inclusive fee of six guineas, have a bath, dinner, and a prostitute.

By this time the Macaronis had arrived, with their breath sweeteners and their perfume. The Macaronis were new only in the degree to which they carried exaggeratedly gentlemanly affectations. Already their predecessors, the beaus, had 'their toilettes set out with washes, perfumes, and cosmetics, and will spend a whole morning in scenting their linen, dressing their hair, and arching their eyebrows'. The Macaronis wore perfume like a badge. Because of this – and because of their fantastic hair styles and elaborate dress – they were labelled homosexual. They were also accused of raping any unprotected woman they came across on the streets at night. One of these accusations must be unfounded.

The Regency bucks who followed the Macaronis reacted against them. Beau Brummell set a fashion of 'studied moderation' in dress and decreed that perfume was 'unnatural' for a man, though he carried cleanliness to almost fetishistic lengths. One man who took Brummell's advice about perfume was the Prince Regent. In 1822, when he was under Brummell's influence, the Prince's perfume bill was £263 for the year. After the two men had fallen out, the bill doubled, to over £500 in 1828.

But the bucks were one thing and ordinary respectable gentlemen another. Most Regency men smelled of Hungary water – still; rose water – still; and eau de Cologne – for a change. Eau de Cologne was particularly popular with men at this period and was used for a variety of purposes – on the flesh, on the clothes, and even as a mouth wash. The playwright Sheridan drank as a cure for his frequent hangovers a mixture of eau de Cologne, brandy, and arbusquade – an antiseptic ointment used on wounds.

Victorian men were scented only indirectly – they smelled mainly of scented linen and of hair oils. When scents for men returned – which was not until after World War II – they came back, via the United States, in disguise. Liquids that were simply toilet waters or light perfumes with a little germicide added were called after-shave lotions. They were given masculine-sounding names like *Tweed*. Mainly they were bought by women and given to their faintly protesting men. But slowly they caught on. Talcum powders for men were marketed. Then the body-splash colognes. Today scents for men are a thriving industry. But we still have a long way to go before we catch up with the ancient Egyptians.

Right: the British boxer Henry Cooper lends his physique and recommendation to *Brut* – a splash-on body lotion for men. Perfumers' advertising agents still feel it necessary to stress that scents are manly – combatting an image of effeminacy that still lingers. It would be a brave man who called Henry Cooper effeminate – he represents the nearest thing we have today to a gladiator of ancient Rome. (The background shows a parade in the arena before a fight between gladiators and wild animals.)

Below: a woman disciple of the Great Beast, Aleister Crowley, shows his mark branded between her breasts. Crowley claimed that his attraction to women was due to an ointment – called the Perfume of Immortality – that he rubbed over his body. It had to be rubbed in so thoroughly, he said, 'that the subtle perfume of the preparation is not detected, or even suspected, by others'. Since it was made of three parts of civet two parts of musk, and one part of ambergris, it is hard to believe that any amount of rubbing in made this a 'subtle' perfume. It was, however, 'a most powerful weapon, the more potent for being secret, against the deepest elements in the nature of those whom it is wished to attract'.

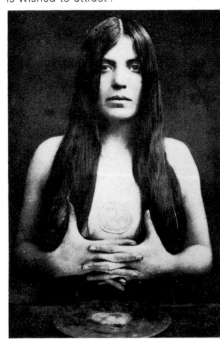

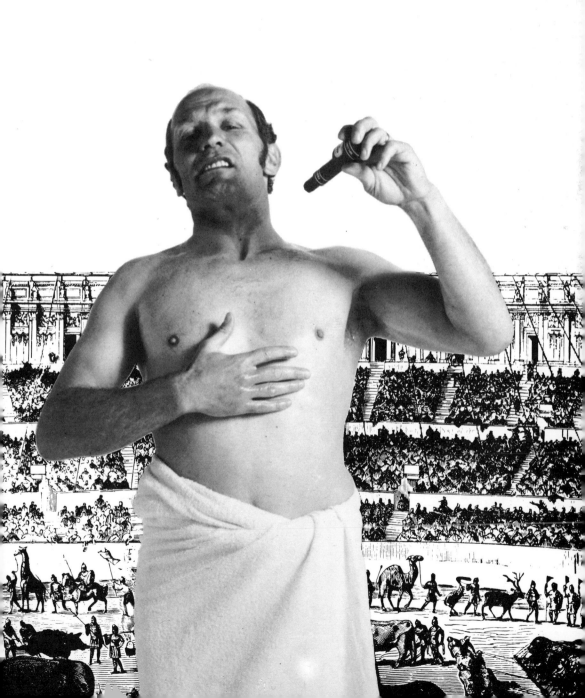

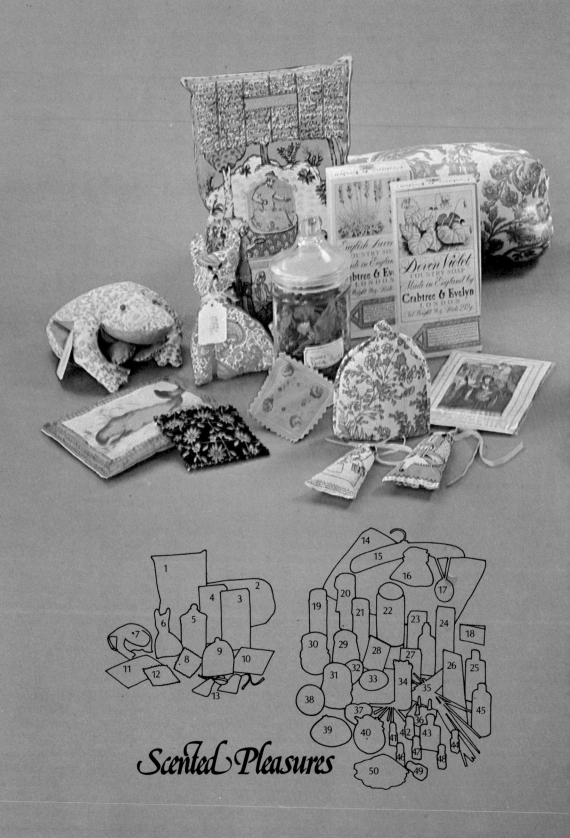

Scented Pleasures

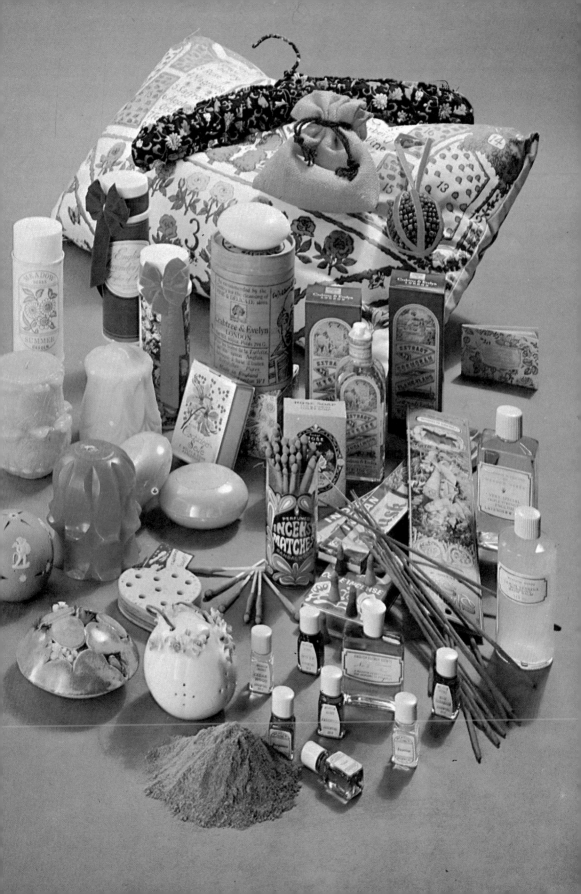

Key to Scented Pleasures
illustrated on the previous page

1 Venetian pot-pourri pillow
2 Pot-pourri of sleep herbs
3 'Devon Violet' country soap
4 'English Lavender' country soap
5 'Royal Roses' pot-pourri
6 'Herbie' cat filled with catmint
7 'Herbie' frog filled with peppermint
8 Patchouli bag for scenting clothes
9 Lemon-verbena egg cosy
10 *Taylor's* 'Cries of London' lavender bag
11 Pot-pourri bag for scenting clothes
12 Lemon verbena bag
13 Lavender dolls
14 Pot-pourri pillow containing sleep herbs
15 Pot-pourri clothes hanger
16 Insect-repellent pot-pourri bag
17 'Elizabethan' cloved orange pomander
18 'Old English' soap leaves for travellers
19 'Summer Garden' hair spray
20 *Taylor of London's* English lavender mist
21 *Taylor of London's* pot-pourri room spray
22 'Old English' flower-scented soap by *Crabtree and Evelyn*
23 *Crabtree and Evelyn's* extract of Mysore sandalwood bath fragrance
24 *Crabtree and Evelyn's* extract of Cormorah ylang-ylang bath fragrance
25 Lavender water
26 Incense sticks
27 Rose soap
28 Orchid soap
29 Jasmine-scented candle
30 Patchouli-scented candle
31 Sandalwood-scented candle
32 and 33 *Jackson's* Redouté rose soap
34 Incense matches
35 Musk-scented incense sticks
36 Self-lighting incense cones
37 Wooden heart-shaped pomander
38 *Wedgwood* pomander
39 Hand-made ceramic pomander
40 Bone-china pomander
41 Essential oil of cedarwood
42 Essential oil of musk
43 *Jackson's* 'Damask Rose' scent
44 Essential oil of rose geranium
45 Lemon-verbena bath balm
46 Essential oil of bergamot
47 Essential oil of patchouli
48 Essential oil of jasmine
49 Essential oil of violet
50 Henna powder

A great deal of flowery language has been expended on the art of the creative perfumer, the man whose job it is to blend a variety of aromas into a new, pleasing, and saleable whole. Writers have tended to compare him to a painter, a poet, or a composer and have been enticed into penning purple passages about his work. Eugene Rimmel, for example, became almost lyrical: 'The first musician who tried to echo with a pierced reed the songs of the birds of the forest, the first painter who attempted to delineate on a polished surface the gorgeous scenes which he beheld around him, were both artists endeavouring to copy nature; and so the perfumer, with a limited number of perfumes at his command, combines them like colours on a palette, and strives to imitate the fragrance of all flowers which are rebellious to his skill, and refuse to yield up their essence. Is he not, then, entitled to claim also the name of an artist, if he approaches even faintly the perfections of his charming models?'

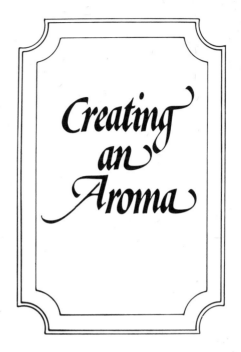

Creating an Aroma

The answer to Rimmel's question has to be an unequivocal 'yes'. The creative perfumer is forced to be an artist. No text book can give the formula for a great painting; no handbook of 'teach-yourself composing' can turn its most diligent reader into another Beethoven. In the end, the painter or the composer is on his own. So is the perfumer. There are no infallible formulae and very few rules of the road for the making of a perfume. It is not even possible to guarantee that, if you mix certain quantities of this with certain quantities of that, you will get at least a not unpleasant smell. You may get a stink instead of a perfume. The trouble is that whenever two aromatic substances are put together they interact, and interact in a largely unpredictable way. Musk plus violet does not, necessarily, equal a scent combining sex and spring so successfully that you market it under the name of *Tonight, Josephine* and make your fortune. More probably, you will have to pour it down the drain and wait for the neighbours to complain. And that is just using two ingredients. Add more, and the element of unpredictability becomes greater.

This is because the perfumer is dealing with immeasurables and intangibles. Take, for example, one simple and common basic ingredient of a perfume, attar of roses. What does the term mean? There are many attars of roses, all different, because every type of rose smells different. The hybrid tea rose Ena Harkness has been described as having 'fruity' overtones; Fragrant Cloud is often described as having an after-taste of cinnamon. This is because no flower scent is a pure, single scent; it is a complexity of scents. What we call 'rose' is dominant, but there are overtones and undertones. It is the blending of these 'tones' that makes a perfume mix so unpredictable.

Already, we have been forced to use metaphors, to speak of 'tones' as though we were discussing a musical

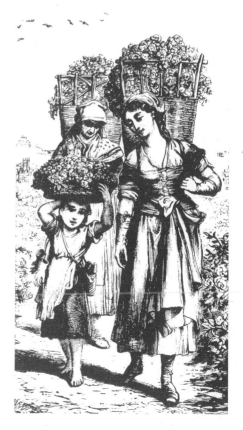

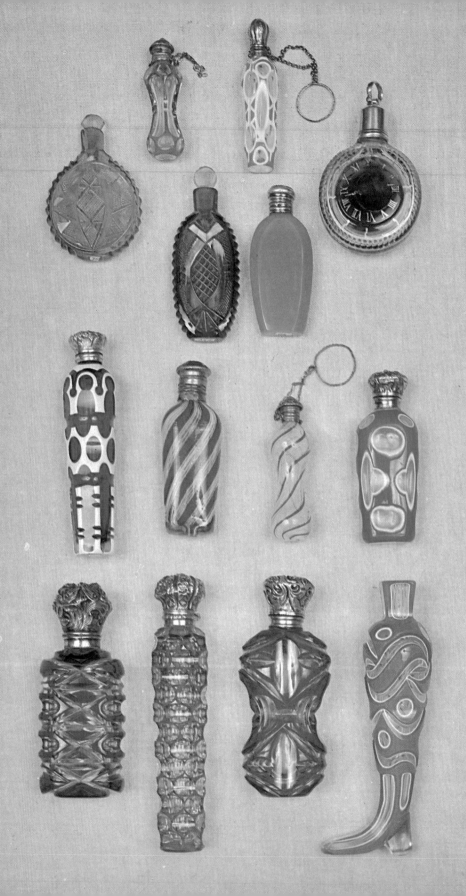

The great age of the scent bottle was the 19th century, when vast numbers were produced in every conceivable shape and in almost every conceivable material. Then, as now, the designer's object was to produce a container that looked expensive, exquisite, and glamorous – in keeping with the image of perfume. Although large scent bottles were made – to contain cologne or toilet water and to stand on the toilet table – the typical Victorian scent bottle was small and handily shaped so that it could be carried in a handbag. It had a constricted neck and small mouth – to reduce the chances of loss by evaporation and to avoid the risk of spillage. It is often hard to distinguish between scent bottles and bottles meant for smelling salts – indeed they were often used interchangeably – and some of the containers shown *left* may have been smelling rather than perfume bottles.

The plainest of the bottles in the illustration – that in blue opaline glass with a silver screw cap – was made in England in about 1880. The clock-faced bottle beside it is of about the same date and is of French manufacture. Its face is a separate layer of blue glass, the numerals are gilt, and the cap is silver gilt. The cut-glass amber-coloured bottles in the top group are earlier. They were made in Bohemia during the first half of the 19th century.

The two centre bottles in the middle row are from the end of the century. The process of twisting different coloured strands into glass was invented by the Venetians, but these bottles were probably made in Stourbridge in England. All the remaining bottles are late 19th-century English; they are made of 'overlay glass'. The pattern is cut through layers of coloured glass to the clear glass beneath.

composition. We are involved in the problem we met in the first chapter, of describing the indescribable. Again we are forced back into analogy. Perhaps the closest comparison we can make is with wines. There is no such thing as port wine, only port wines. And we have to talk of the 'bouquet' of wines, meaning those intangible subtleties that make one wine differ from another. The problems are very similar. Although we may happen to like both claret and burgundy, we are not likely to create our ideal wine by mixing equal quantities of the two together.

So why mix at all? Why not be content with a single fragrance? There are several answers to these questions. One is that the perfumer is in business to make a profit; he has to have a product that is different from his rivals. Another is that there is no such thing as a standard, consistent, single scent. Yet another is that a perfume has to have certain qualities, such as stability and staying power, that can be achieved only by mixing. So it is not just a matter of extracting the perfume of, say, the rose, bottling it, marketing it, and managing without the creative perfumer. Apart from anything else, undiluted single scents are unlikely to be all-time best sellers. By themselves, and in bulk, they have a singularly overpowering and unpleasant smell.

The perfumer, then, is forced to be a mixer. When Rimmel wrote, the perfumer had at his disposal some 500 fragrant ingredients, all of them natural products – essential oils, gums, and flower and fruit extracts. Today, he has about 4,000 materials available. In practical, business terms, this reduces to about two or three hundred most-used substances. With these the perfumer concocts his new perfume. He works by guesswork, rather like a small boy with a new chemistry set. It is experienced, educated, and skilled guesswork, but guesswork none the less.

It may take years to perfect a new perfume. Surrounded by as many bottles as a pharmacist, each containing an essential oil or scent, the perfumer begins his blending. He starts, of course, with an idea, or a theme. He has a shrewd idea of what he is aiming at and he knows the main aromas he will use. But from then on he is as pragmatic as a politician. As he adds perhaps a touch of jasmine to give 'smoothness', or the merest drop of musk to add 'excitement', he tests continually. He dips small strips of blotting paper, known as *mouillettes,* into the mixture, lays them aside to dry, and sniffs them to see how close he is coming to his final target. Appropriately, he is known in the trade as a 'nose'.

The blending takes so long because the new perfume has to be both attractive and distinctive and because it has to be tested under a variety of conditions. The most beautiful perfume is useless if it will not last for several hours when worn. It is useless if its aroma changes in the course of time, or with varying conditions of heat and humidity. It is useless if it does not smell at dawn the same as it does at dusk. Most important of all it must give off, throughout its life, a consistent aroma.

A fine perfume is rather like a three-course meal. It gives off first the hors d'oeuvre, known as its topnote. This is the first scent that hits the nose as soon as the stopper is removed from the bottle. Often it is a 'light' aroma, perhaps lemon or bergamot, which fades fairly quickly. Then comes the main course, the heart or the theme of the perfume. Finally, for dessert, the perfume gives off its endnote, the fall that gives it its characteristic, individual flavour.

An important part of any perfume is its fixative. This is the ingredient that gives the perfume its permanence, ensuring that its varying ingredients do not evaporate at different rates and so in time change the nature of the perfume. The skill of a 'nose' is perhaps best displayed in his ability to handle the fixative. Different types of perfumes need different types of fixatives. A heavy fixative may overpower a delicate scent. And the problem is that every fixative is itself an aromatic substance, which will change the nature of the perfume like any other ingredient.

Most perfumes – even the most expensive – contain a high proportion of synthetic materials. It has been calculated that two thirds of the raw materials used in perfumery today are synthetic. This is partly because the cost of the natural products has become prohibitive. In 1974 natural musk absolute cost the manufacturing perfumer £1,525 a kilo; the best attar of roses, from Bulgaria, was £1,900 a kilo; and violet-leaf absolute was £1,250 a kilo. Jasmine absolute cost £150 a kilo, and even lavender absolute was £30. Another reason is that there is a shortage of the natural product. Two tons of roses, or a hundred million petals, are needed to produce one pound of attar of roses. It is rather like refining gold from low-grade ore. Yet not only the perfumers, but also the soap-flake and detergent producers, measure their consumption of perfume ingredients in thousands of tons a year.

There are two groups of synthetic aromatics: those that are copies of natural products and those that are not only man-made but man-invented. These are the scents that do not exist in nature but are now part of the perfumer's armoury. Some of the most sophisticated 'modern' perfumes could not have existed without artificial chemicals, in particular that group of chemicals called aldehydes.

Synthetics are not necessarily cheaper than natural products, but they can be produced in large quantities. Neither are they necessarily inferior to the natural products; it isn't possible to say that a 'natural' perfume is 'better' than a synthetic one. On the whole, synthetics are more consistent and more predictable than nature's scents, and it could be argued that they are therefore likely to give consistently better results. On the other

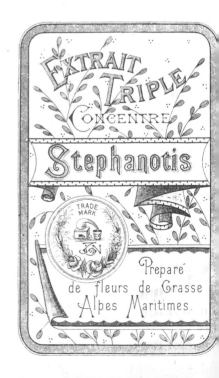

EXTRAIT TRIPLE CONCENTRÉ

Stephanotis

TRADE MARK

Préparé de fleurs de Grasse Alpes Maritimes.

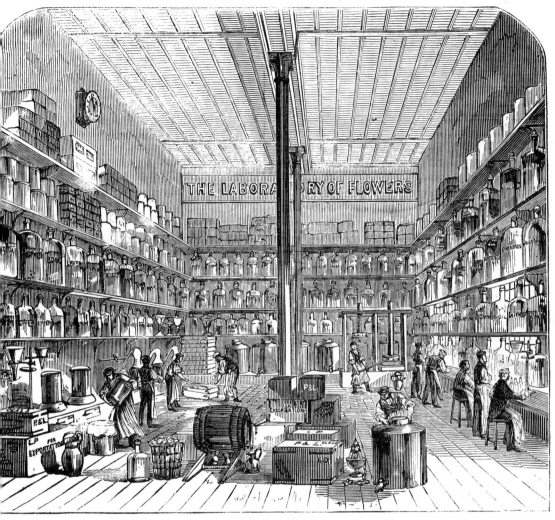

MESSRS. PIESSE AND LUBIN'S PERFUME MANUFACTORY,
IN THE ST. KATHERINE'S DOCKS.

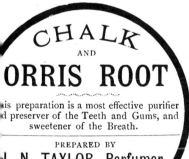

CHALK
AND
ORRIS ROOT

is preparation is a most effective purifier
d preserver of the Teeth and Gums, and
sweetener of the Breath.

PREPARED BY

J. N. TAYLOR, Perfumer,
—67—
Mortimer Street,
Regent Street, London, W.

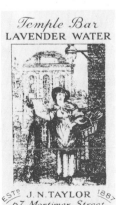

Temple Bar
LAVENDER WATER

J. N. TAYLOR
67, Mortimer Street,
London. W. I.

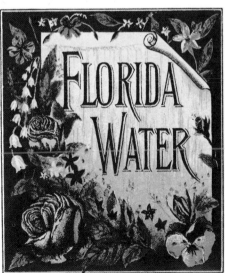

FLORIDA WATER

On this page, and on pages 118 and 121, are shown some of the
scent labels used by one London manufacturer over the
past 50 years.

hand, traditionalists in the perfume world are still heard to mutter into their beards that synthetics lack the 'warmth' of naturals.

One of the first perfumes to use synthetic ingredients was *Chanel No. 5*, one of the all-time classics of perfumery, which was blended by Ernst Beaux in 1923. Coty's *L'Aimant* and Lanvin's *Arpège* followed within a few years. Both used synthetics; both became classics.

The use of synthetics has caused problems of description. Many fragrances that are now manufactured artificially are still being sold under the names of the natural products they resemble. This may be permissible, or at least understandable. Any advertising agent might be forgiven for preferring not to offer a waiting world a perfume called *Hydroxycitronellal*; oil of dew-drenched lilies of the valley sounds far more romantic. But the result is that it is almost impossible for the buyer to know what he is getting.

This applies even to the so-called single-note 'natural' scents now enjoying a vogue – the liquids sold as musk, patchouli, amber, and sandalwood, for example. All of these, of necessity, contain a high proportion of synthetic materials. What these synthetics are depends upon the taste, experience, and honesty of the perfumer, as well as the price bracket within which he is working. Consequently, Smith's brand of sandalwood will smell very different from Brown's, and Jones's musk will be totally unlike Green's. Neither will smell like natural musk or sandalwood.

Perfumers have always been understandably secretive about their formulae and have described their products only in the most general terms. Yardley's *Khadine* – 'sophisticated, soft and haunting, offering excitement and femininity in the same breath' – is a blend of spices of clove and pepper, attar of rose, jasmine, lily of the valley, sandalwood, vetivert, and patchouli. Nina Ricci's *Farouche* – 'seductive without being suggestive, sensuous without being sensational' – is a blend of jasmine, rose absolute, 'rare fruits of the Orient, woodsy blossoms . . . a hundred precious ingredients'. Elizabeth Arden's *Blue Grass* – 'inspired by the freshness of a summer's day' – mingles 'jasmine, geranium, roses and lilies of the valley with other fragrant blossoms. Crisp touches of lavender and an underlying base of green moss add a cooling note.' It is all very different from the details on the label of a sauce bottle.

The reason is, of course, that the perfumer is in a highly competitive business. His perfume has to be different, has to be uncopiable, and, preferably, inimitable. It also has to anticipate, or at least keep up with, trends in public likes and dislikes. There has recently been a citrus trend, during which the fragrances of lemon, lime, orange, and bergamot have been popular. Lemon scent, in particular, has marked a gamut of products – from the whole range of Love cosmetics, through Colgate's *Fresh* soap, to a furniture polish,

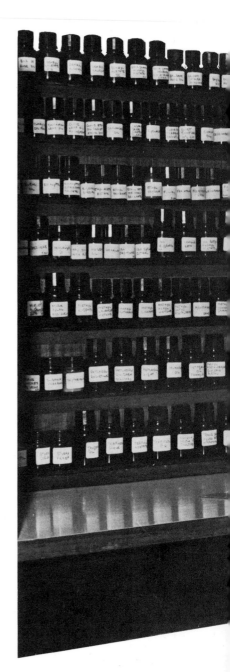

A perfumer composes a fragrance at her 'organ', the research bench at which she works in the scent manufacturer's laboratory. Its 'keyboard' is the rows of shelves that bring easily to her hand the raw materials used in the creation of a blended perfume.

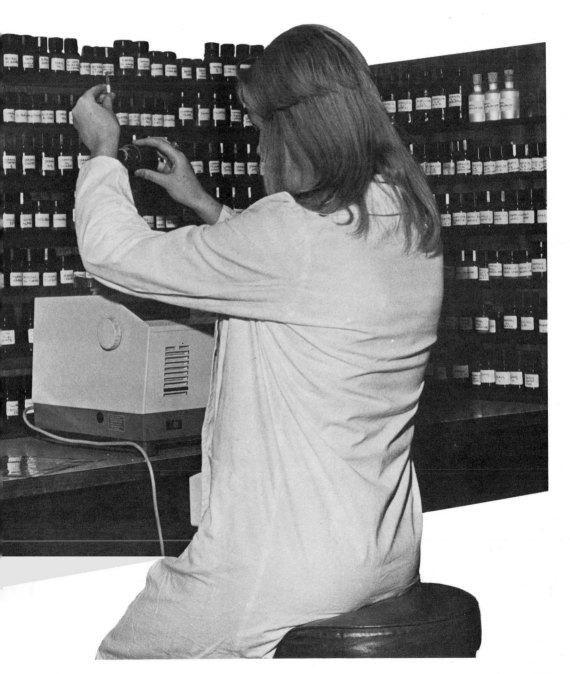

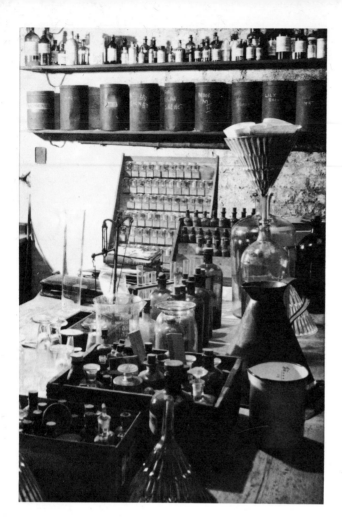

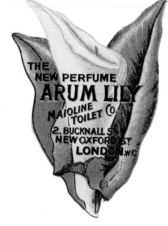

Left: a photograph, taken in 1963, showing a corner of Taylor of London's perfumery shop in Mortimer Street. The simple chemists' vessels, scales, stoppered jars, and labelled canisters for storing finished sachet mixtures demonstrate the reliance of the business on traditional, hand methods of manufacture.

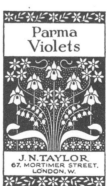

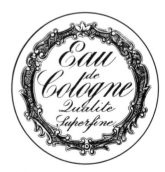

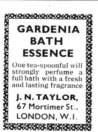

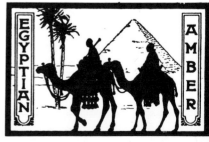

Johnson's *Lemon Sparkle*. Apparently now replacing citrus are what are known as 'green-note' perfumes – those with fragrances reminiscent of crushed pea pods, plant stems, and leaves. Molineux's *Vivre* and Estée Lauder's *Alliage* are examples. Flower perfumes, particularly single-note flower fragrances, have also had a rebirth of popularity. A number of perfume manufacturers have brought out sophisticated new perfumes with a strong floral note. *Chanel No. 19*, based on violets, is one.

Green-note and single-floral scents are part of the back-to-nature movement in perfumery, which has been the most outstanding trend in recent years. This has become involved with the craze for buying concentrated perfume essences and wearing them either singly or blended in different, experimental proportions. One firm offers a whole range of essences including patchouli, musk, jasmine, mandarin, verbena, and sandalwood. In fact most of these essences are synthetic and to that extent a fraud. Still, pure natural essence of musk would certainly be too unpleasant to use.

These essences have been a commercial success because they have been taken up by the young – who, as a rule, do not buy traditional complex perfumes. They have, however, accepted simple essences, and the hippy sub-culture of the young is now so well-established, and has so much money to spend, that it can support a commercial structure dependent upon supplying its status symbols. Essential oils are part of the status product mix, along with Moroccan clothes, Turkish brass, Tarot cards, and incense.

It is perfectly possible to be a do-it-yourself perfumer using these packaged essential oils. Better still, there is

Below: sorting roses for making perfume – Grasse, France, 1891.

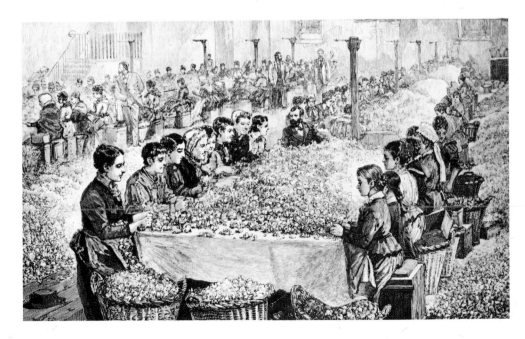

already on the market a kit containing all the ingredients – including fixative and base – a home perfumer needs. Or you can make your own perfume from natural floral ingredients. You will be rather limited, the process is a long and tedious one, and you are not likely to produce a breathtakingly classic perfume, but it can be done.

In a quart of water dissolve a teaspoonful of alum. Boil three quarters of a pound of animal fat and a quarter of pound of lard in the alum water. When all the fat has dissolved, strain the liquid through muslin into a basin and let it cool. The fat will come to the surface and solidify. Separate it from the liquid, melt it down again, pour it, equally divided, into two shallow dishes, and let it solidify again.

Go into the garden and pick two good handfuls of fresh, unbruised petals, choosing any flowers whose scent attracts you. Spread the petals an inch or so thick over the fat in one dish and invert the other on top of it, so that you have a fat-and-petal sandwich. Leave for 48 hours. Then throw away the petals, go out and pick some more, and put the fresh petals into the sandwich. Go on changing the petals every second day for about a month. By this time the fat will be saturated with petal fragrance. Scrape it into a screw-top jar and add to it an equal volume of spirits of wine. Screw down the top and place the jar in a dark cupboard. Shake it well at least once a day. Do this for a couple of months. Then strain the liquid through muslin into a suitable container and put it on the dressing table. You have, with any luck, made a light floral perfume.

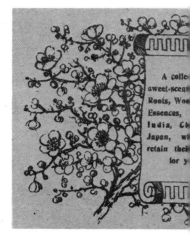

A colle[...]
sweet-scen[...]
Roots, Woo[...]
Essences,
India, Ch[...]
Japan, w[...]
retain thei[...]
for y[...]

There are easier and more certain ways. One, of course, is to buy a do-it-yourself liquid perfume kit. Another is to forget about liquid perfume and make a pot-pourri – that is, a mixture of flower petals, herbs, and spices that, in a suitable container, gives off its scent to the room, cupboard, or wardrobe in which it is placed. The pot-pourri may be put in any open bowl, when it will look attractive as well as smell sweet, or in a pomander, when it will retain its fragrance for a very much longer period.

Pot-pourris have been used since medieval times, when they were made from herbs and wild flowers. Later on, they were made from flowers picked from cottage gardens. Today, pot-pourris have become popular again – at London's Heathrow airport they are the second biggest attraction, next only to wines and spirits, to tourists and travellers. But garden flowers today have lost much of their scent, mainly through intensive breeding for bigger and shapelier blossoms and through hybridization. So modern pot-pourris usually have to be strengthened with essential oils.

Nothing much has changed over the centuries in the commercial manufacture of pot-pourris. They still have to be made by cottage-industry methods. The petals are too fragile to be mixed by machine. Wooden rakes and spoons with rounded edges are still the only tools that can safely be used on them. The spices are still hand-ground in a china pestle with a china mortar. The petals, spices, and oils are still mixed together on a wooden table – usually made of teak, because teak is the only wood so hard that it absorbs none of the essential oils. Even the packing has to be done by hand. Consequently, commercial pot-pourri making has remained in the hands of a few traditional suppliers – all of whom jealously guard their trade secrets.

Like the perfume manufacturers, the pot-pourri makers have, because of the increasing demand for their product, problems with the supply of their raw materials. Commercial production in this country relies almost exclusively on imported petals – since our climate and relatively short growing season make it difficult to guarantee flowers of consistent quality and quantity. Rose petals, for example, are imported mainly from Morocco, Turkey, and Persia; lavender comes from Grasse and other parts of the south of France; jasmine has to be brought from Italy and patchouli from India. The spices, too, come from all over the world – vanilla from Malagasy, cloves from Zanzibar. Even so, there is now a world-wide shortage of raw materials.

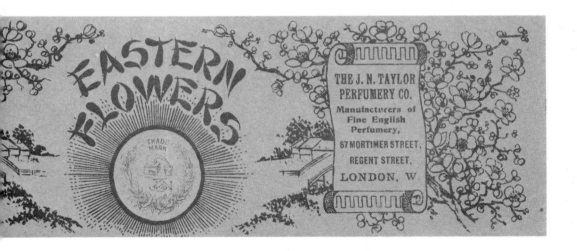

Very adequate pot-pourris can, however, be made at home. There are two ways of doing this. One is to buy the dried petals and essences by mail order, so that the only task is the mixing. This is a method increasingly used in schools, many of which have begun to teach the art of pot-pourri making. Another way is to begin at the beginning and collect the petals from your own and your friends' gardens.

On the next two pages we list, in table form, suitable ingredients for a home-made pot-pourri, and give one simple pot-pourri recipe that makes use of ingredients selected from these tables.

Common Ingredients used in Pot-Pourri Making

Table A
ESSENTIAL FLOWERS
Roses
Lavender

Table B
MISCELLANEOUS INGREDIENTS
Orris root
Sea salt
Lemon peel
Orange peel

Table C
LESS ESSENTIAL FLOWERS
Acacia blossom
Carnations
Clover
Delphiniums
Elder
Geraniums
Heliotrope
Jonquil
Lemon blossom
Lilac
Lilies of the Valley
Lime
Mallow
Marigolds
Meadow Sweet
Mignonette
Narcissus
Orange blossom
Pinks
Verbascum
Violets
Wallflowers

*for colour only

Table D
SCENTED LEAVES/HERBS
Angelica
Bay
Laurel
Lemon balm
Mint
Rosemary
Tarragon
Thyme

Table E
GROUND SPICES
Allspice
Cinnamon
Cloves
Mace
Nutmegs

Table F
OILS
Almond
Bergamot
Cedarwood
Geranium
Jasmine
Lavender
Lemon Grass
Lemon Verbena
Neroli
Patchouli
Rose
Sandalwood
Vetivert
Violet

Table G
FOR MOISTENING DRY POT-POURRIS
Brandy
Eau de Cologne
Rose water
Lemon juice

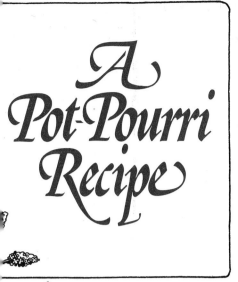

A Pot-Pourri Recipe

from Table A	1 lb. Rose Petals – 1 lb. Lavender
from Table B	¼ lb Orris Root – ½ lb. Sea Salt
from Tables C+D	¼ lb Mixed Flowers ¼ lb Mixed Scented leaves + herbs
from Table E	1 oz. Cinnamon – 1 oz. Cloves – 1 oz. Allspice
from Table F	½ oz. Neroli – ½ oz. Lemon Grass ½ oz. Lavender – ½ oz. Geranium

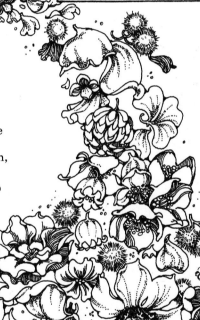

Make your pot-pourri in this way:

Gather your rose petals, preferably in the early morning just after the dew has dried from them.

Pick the lavender and the flowers, leaves, and herbs.

Lay out everything you have harvested to dry. Keep the rose petals and the lavender separate from each other and from the other ingredients. All the petals, flowers, leaves, and herbs should be spread on to pieces of paper and left to dry in the sun, in an airing cupboard, or in a dry room.

When everything is thoroughly dry – petals should be as crisp as cornflakes – mix together the orris root and sea salt. Take any airtight container – a screw-top jar is ideal – and put a layer of rose petals in the bottom. Sprinkle on top of this a layer of salt-orris mixture. Continue making alternate layers of salt-orris and petals until the container is full.

Seal the container and keep it in a dark, dry place for seven to ten days. Stir the contents thoroughly as often as you can, at least once a day.

Now mix the spices and oils together in a bowl and add this blend to the lavender. The lavender flowers will absorb the oil so that it does not stain the flower petals. Then add the rose petals and other flowers, leaves, and herbs.

Stir and re-heap the mound at least once a day for several days. Then put it into a tightly covered container and leave it to mature for three or four weeks.

Your pot-pourri is now ready to be put into pomanders or open dishes. Keep the stock of pot-pourri sealed in its container; you will need it to refill the pomanders. Make sure that the pot-pourri in use never gets too dry. Moisten it whenever necessary with a little brandy or, if you prefer, a mixture of eau de Cologne, brandy, and lemon juice.

We have given just one recipe, but a variety of pot-pourris may be made by selecting from the ingredients in the tables. There are very few hard and fast rules in pot-pourri making. It is, however, essential that any petals, leaves, or herbs are absolutely dry – otherwise the pot-pourri will smell musty. It is advisable always to incorporate roses and lavender, although the proportions of each may be varied. Roses, though, should always account for about half the total bulk of all the petals, herbs, and leaves used. The orris root and sea salt mixture described in our recipe is desirable if not essential. Orris root is a fixative; it makes the pot-pourri last longer. Dried lemon and orange peel are optional extras; they may be included at Step 6. Any of the fragrant flowers listed in Table C will give good results, although marigold and mallow add little to the perfume; they are included for colour only. There is no reason why you should not use musk and other essential oils referred to elsewhere in this book, but, if you do use animal oils, use them sparingly.

There are short cuts to pot-pourri making. Instead of picking and drying your own flowers and herbs, you can buy ready-dried flower mixtures from certain specialist shops – such as, in London, Jacksons of Piccadilly – and mail order houses. You may then use either the 'wet' method or the 'dry' method of making your pot-pourri.

The wet method uses pot-pourri oil. Several manufacturers sell oil formulations which are a blend of traditional scented ingredients. They are often sold as 'pot-pourri revivers', because their main function is to freshen up pot-pourris that have lost their smell. All you have to do is add the reviver to the lavender as in Step 6 in our recipe, and carry on from there.

The dry method uses pot-pourri powder, which takes the effort and the gamble out of pot-pourri making. The powder is a mixture of ground spices, fixatives, and essential oils. The procedure is very simple. Just mix the powder thoroughly with your dried flowers and follow Step 7.

The term 'dry pot-pourri' is perhaps deceptive. No pot-pourri mixture is dry enough to use in a sachet to perfume linen. Sachets can, however, be made at home – although the choice of ingredients is limited because few flowers retain their fragrance when dehydrated. But roses, lavender, and most garden herbs may be used.

The renewed popularity of sachets and pot-pourris is just one sign of a new realization in the 1970s that our surroundings, as well as our persons, can be made pleasanter by being scented. Or, in the words – even more appropriate in our polluted age – of the 17th-century versifier Abraham Cowley:

Who that has reason, and his smell,
Would not among roses and jasmine dwell,
Rather than all his spirits choke
With exhalations of dirt and smoke?

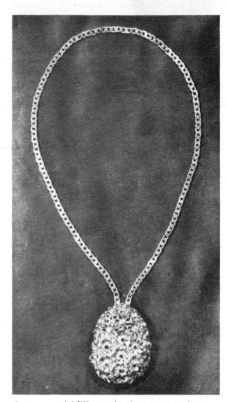

Above: gold filigree locket pomander made by Asprey's for Taylor of London – valued in 1974 at about £1,500.

Below: pierced soft metal pomander with painted flowers, manufactured in about 1909 and probably of German origin.

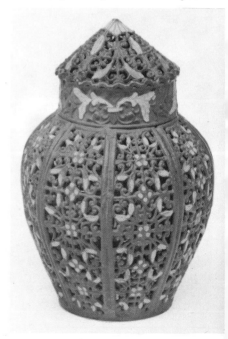

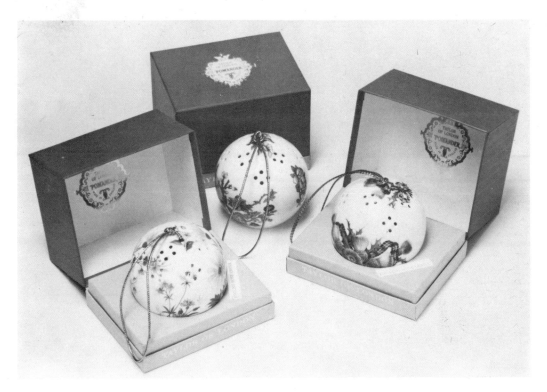

Above: selection of English bone-china pomanders.

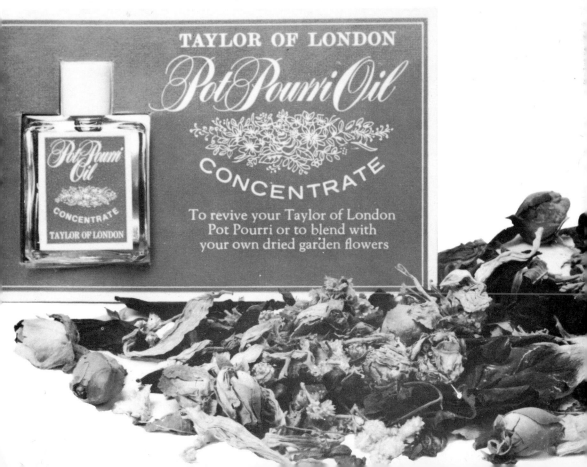

ACKNOWLEDGEMENTS

Aldus Archives 40(B); Art Gallery of New South Wales, Sydney (Edward Poynter, British 1836-1919, *The Visit of the Queen of Sheba to King Solomon,* Oil on canvas 231 × 350.4cm) 68-69; Photos Ashmolean Museum 9(T), 45(T), 82; Reproduced by permission of the Trustees of the British Library 38; J. Allan Cash 21(T); after Arthur Mee, *Children's Encyclopaedia,* Cassell & Co. Limited 70-71; City of Manchester Art Galleries 100-101(T); By kind permission of Henry Cooper and Fabergé 107(CB); *Daily Telegraph Colour Library* 60, 61; Mary Evans Picture Library 18(B), 19, 27(T), 30, 33(B), 37, 43, 46, 48, 52, 58(T), 64, 67, 88, 90, 93, 115; Werner Forman 20(T), 21(B), 28, 29; Guildhall Library, City of London 72-73; Houbigant 89; Courtesy I.F.F. (Great Britain) Ltd. 116-117; Courtesy Jacksons of Piccadilly 108-109; Kobal Collection 22(T); Mansell Collection 8(T), 26, 27 (B), 44, 45(B), 51, 55(B), 62-63, 78, 83, 86, 87(B), 92, 94-95, 96, 98(B), 101(B); after Mansell 12-13, 41B; Photo Meyer 49; ©Parkshot Paper Products Mfg. Ltd. 10, 108-109, 116-117, (Marilyn Day) 6, 8-9, 11, 16, 31(B), 33(T), 36, 40(T), 45(T), 58(B), 66-67, 122-123, (Peter Dennis) 41, 70-71, 75, 98(T), (Tony Morris) 34, 50, 55(T); after Picturepoint, London 36; Mauro Pucciarelli, Rome 56-57; Radio Times Hulton Picture Library 16, 31(T), 35, 39(B), 59, 79, 84, 85, 87(T), 91, 103, 106, 107 (background), 111; Ronan Picture Library 42, 47, 66(T), 102(T), 119; R. S. Skelton 32; Courtesy of Sotheby's Belgravia 24-25, 97, 104-105; Spectrum Colour Library 53, 65; *The Sunday Times* 23, 80; Courtesy Taylor of London 2-3, 114, 115, 118, 121, 124, 125; Victoria & Albert Museum, London 31(B), 76-77, (Photo R. B. Fleming ©Aldus Books) 17; by kind permission of Edmund Launert and Walsall Lithographic Co. Ltd. 112; G. Heil/ZEFA 20(B).

The author wishes to give special thanks to his designer John Watson, A.R.C.A. He is indebted also, for help and information, to: Michael Stewart-Smith and Miss Grace Garner of Taylor of London; David Butterfield of I.F.F.; Francis Fitt of Jacksons of Piccadilly; and Arthur J. McCarthy of V. Berg & Sons Limited.